Psychological Aspects in time of Pandemic

Juan Moisés de la Serna

Translated by Jacqueline Passfield

Tektime Editorial

2020

"Psychological Aspects in time of Pandemic"

Written by Juan Moisés de la Serna

Translated by Jacqueline Passfield

1st edition: November 2020

Distributed by Tektime

Prologue

In light of the very positive reception to the article entitled "Cual es el papel del psicólogo ante el nuevo Coronavirus (COVID-19)?" ("What is the role of psychology in the face of the new Coronavirus (COVID-19)?") published in La Cátedra Abierta de Psicología y Neurosciencias on 12th February 2020, and the general interest evoked amongst fellow psychologists and other people with an interest in psychology, I have decided to produce this book, which addresses the subject of the psychological perspective in times of a pandemic.

Despite the fact that information concerning health crises such as COVID-19 is very recent and in some cases quite changeable, I am going to present a work based on current data sourced principally from scientific publications, and which will include, from the same sources, statements from various experts.

A book accessible to all who wish to delve into the psychological aspects of a mass phenomenon in times of a health crisis, as in the case of COVID-19.

Dedicated to my parents

INDEX

Chapter 1: Introduction to COVID-19

One may speak of a personal or a social crisis. A personal crisis takes place when an internal or external circumstance occurs which changes the manner in which an individual perceives their own present, future and even past, making them question either their own role in life, or all their thoughts and beliefs up to that particular moment. Such is the case when a family member, particularly a close one, dies, or an accident occurs, with associated health or autonomy implications. One may also face a crisis due to emotional issues, such as the breakdown of a relationship, or the divorce of one's parents as a teenager. From a psychological perspective, such crises are viewed as being caused by the effect of many different circumstances upon an individual. But then there are the social crises, as in the cases of humanitarian crises, where millions of people abandon all they have and flee towards an uncertain future. Likewise, economic crises, where thousands of people lose their jobs overnight and with them their incomes, putting both their own survival and those of their loved ones at risk (@NTN24ve, 2018) (See Illustration 1).

Included in this type of crisis are those related to health, in which a disease may put at risk the life of an individual who, a few days earlier was perfectly healthy.

Pandemics and health emergencies may be included in this category, as in the case of COVID-19, a disease that has mobilized thousands of doctors and health personnel who struggle daily, even risking their own lives, in mitigating the effects of the virus,

NTN24 Venezuela
@NTN24ve

Venezuela entra en la lista de países con crisis humanitaria encabezada por África bit.ly/2xSr9iw

VENEZUELA ENTRE LOS PAÍSES CON LAS CRISIS HUMANITARIAS MÁS DESATENDIDAS DEL MUNDO
1. República Democrática del Congo
2. Sudán del Sur
3. República Centroafricana
4. Burundi
5. Etiopía
6. Palestina
7. Myanmar
8. Yemen
9. Venezuela
10. Nigeria
NTN24 VENEZUELA
Fuente: Consejo Noruego de Refugiados

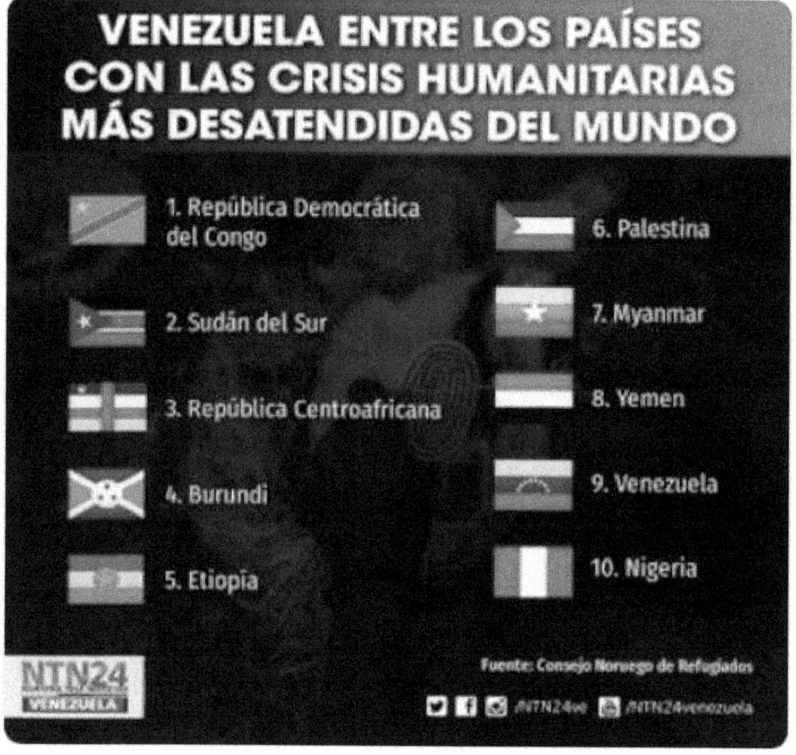

12:45 a. m. · 10 jun. 2018 · TweetDeck

Illustration 1. Tweet – Humanitarian Crisis

[Venezuela enters the list of countries with humanitarian crises, headed by Africa]

Whilst the media often affords the most visibility to numbers of cases and deaths, such information being provided from different governments and the webpage of the WHO (World Health Organisation), the Center for Systems Science and Engineering at John Hopkins University, USA (John Hopkins, CSSE, 2020) reports, numerically and visually, the numbers of cases, deaths and recoveries, both for each individual country and worldwide.

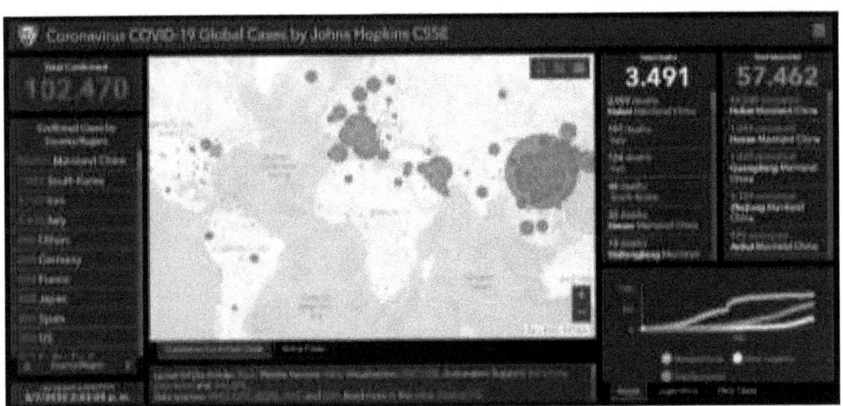

Illustration 2. Infections as at 7th March 2020

Thus, on 7th March 2020, which is when this book begins, the number of cases worldwide is 102.470, distributed amongst 101 countries. China has 80,651 cases, followed by South Korea with 7,041 and Iran with 4,747. Spain is in tenth position with 401 cases (See Illustration

2).

The portal also reports that the number of deaths to date is 3,491 people, with 57,462 having recovered from the disease.

Updating the previous data on 19th March 2020, the number affected worldwide is 218,827 people, distributed amongst 160 countries, with the number of worldwide deaths 8,811. (See Illustration 3)

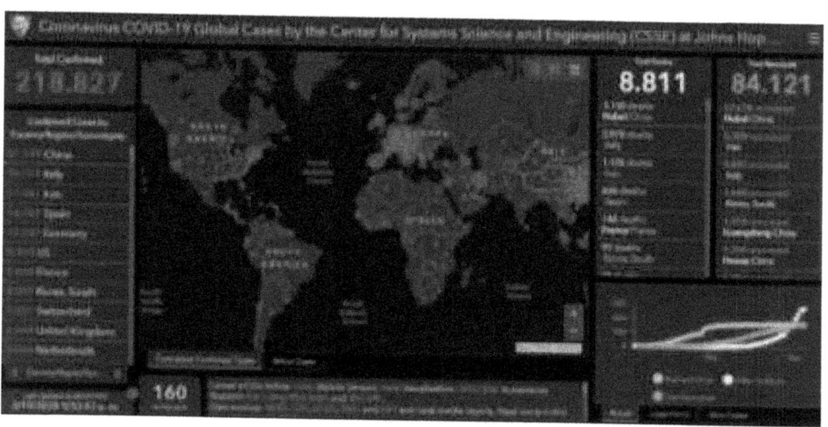

Illustration 3. Infections as at 19th March 2020

Looking at Google (Google Trend, 2020) regarding the search trends for COVID-19, a term designated by the WHO on 11th February 2020 to refer to the new coronavirus that emerged in a province of China, and whose first case of the disease was reported on 31st December 2019 (WHO, 2020), it can be seen how numbers of searches for this term have been progressively increasing worldwide, doubling between 11th and 12th February, 23rd and 24th February and 1st and 2nd March, a reduction only observed between 28th February to March 1st (See Illustration 4).

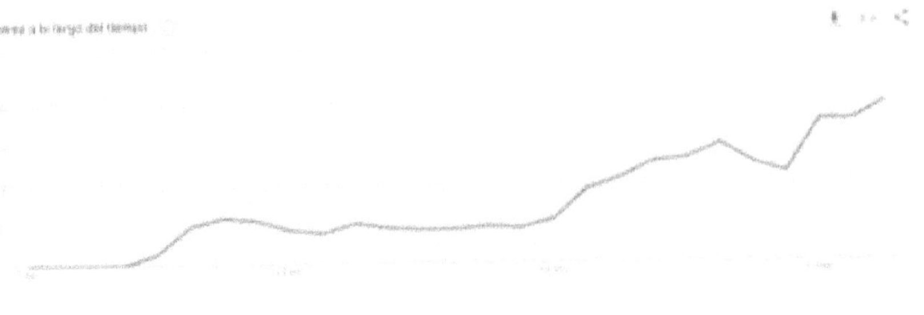

Illustration 4. Evolution of the search term

Regarding interest shown by specific countries, it can be seen that the country that has generated most searches within the last month has been Singapore, followed by Iceland, China and Hong Kong. Out of the total 65 countries in Google's results, USA is in 20th position and Spain is 48th. Turkey is in final position (See Illustration 5).

As can be seen, there is no direct correspondence between the countries with the greatest number of cases and the concern generated amongst their populations reflected in the searches. This may be due to other factors, such as the generation of alarmism in certain populations for instance, or usage of means other than Google to obtain pertinent information. For example, in some Asian countries the most commonly used search engine is Baidu.

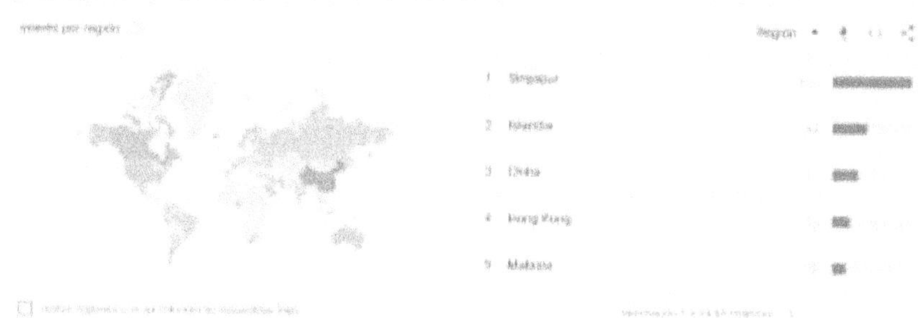

Illustration 5. Searches by country

It should also be noted that COVID-19 was previously referred to as the new coronavirus 2019 (n-CoV) and also known as "China virus" or "Wuhan virus" – Wuhan being the name of the Chinese province where the virus originated, so some users will continue to search with these old terms. In addition, the term 'coronavirus', which is the name of the family of this particular virus, or simply 'virus' may be used. For this reason, if data is only collected for the term 'COVID-19' the overview would be incomplete. This could explain the difference demonstrated between countries in terms of number of deaths and order of interest shown from Google searches.

Therefore, if the previous search is carried out, but including the terms COVID, Virus and Coronavirus as search terms, it can be seen that concern for this issue began on 20th January 2020, and that the term COVID or

COVID-19, which is its official name, is hardly used at all in information searches on the subject, with the search of the term Virus being considerably higher and the term Coronavirus higher still (See Illustration 6).

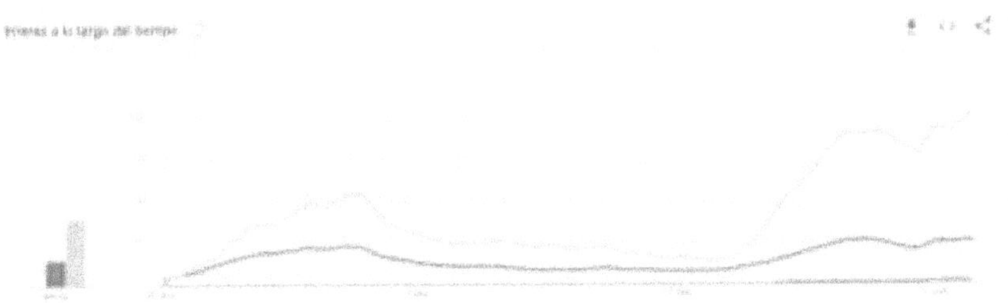

Illustration 6. Terms on Google related to COVID

In the previous graph one can see there was initial interest shown in both terms Virus and Coronavirus between 20th and 31st January followed by a progressive loss of interest up until 20th February when interest in the term Coronavirus increases exponentially.

Focussing on this last term, the country that has searched it the most on Google is Italy, followed by Singapore and Switzerland. Out of the 64 countries for which data is available Spain is in fifth place and USA is nineteenth (See Illustration 7).

This data does correspond to the growing number of infections, except in the case of Ireland where one could speak of an instance of social alarmism over actual data of the time.

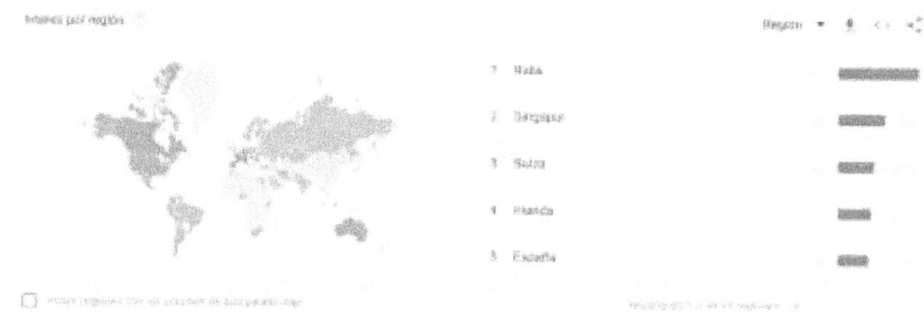

Illustration 7. Search of the term Coronavirus by country

The name of COVID-19

One of the problems facing social psychologists is in achieving customer brand loyalty, a brand being that which is used in the identification of a certain person, product or company. Normally when thinking of a company like Coca-Cola, McDonald's or IKEA, it is with reference to the products they sell. With other brands such as UPS, Iberia or Microsoft, it is with regards the services they offer. This is something which exerts a decisive influence on the purchase of any product or service, which is no longer based just on one's own judgement, but on the influence of the opinion of others and the media via advertising.

If one thinks of Stephen Hawking, Barack Obama or Rafael Nadal in the same way, it is no longer in terms of products or services, but in respect of their personal branding or brand they have developed through their scientific, political and sporting careers respectively. In other words, emotional aspects become associated with a brand which may be linked to a person, a company and even a place.

The same happens when it comes to the naming of disasters, as in the case of the tropical cyclones which annually afflict a large part of the Caribbean and North

America. According to the World Meteorological Organization (WMO, 2020) these names follow pre-established rotating lists, and for many they leave behind the memories of the effects of Hurricane Katrina in 2005 or Ike in 2008.

In principle the names bear no relation to the dates of the events, the damaging incidents themselves, or the most affected areas. Amongst them are English and Spanish names e.g. Barry, Gonzalo and they may be male or female e.g. Lorenzo, Laura. But does the name of a tropical cyclone have any impact upon the population?

An answer to this question has been sought by the Department of Administration and Business in conjunction with the Department of Psychology, the Institute of Communications Research, and the Women and Gender Surveys Research Laboratory of the University of Illinois; together with the Department of Statistics of Arizona State University (Jung, Shavitt, Viswanathan & Hilbe, 2014).

The study analysed the climatic consequences of hurricanes in the USA over the last six decades, differentiating between those with male and female names. The first finding was that those with female names had been the most destructive and the cause of most deaths.

It should be remembered that the list of names is preassigned and their assignment organised consecutively, so a priori there is no relationship between the gender of the name and the intensity of the hurricane. A list of hurricane names, 5 male and 5 female were given to 346 participants for them to rate the considered extent of each hurricane's intensity on a Likert-type scale from 1 – 7. The results showed that male-named hurricanes tend to be evaluated as more destructive than female-named hurricanes, regardless of each participant's gender.

This study made it possible to understand why, in the face of warnings from the authorities, sometimes more and sometimes fewer preventative measures tend to be taken. It is, in fact, simply due to whether the hurricane's assigned name is male or female.

In contrast, the designation of diseases within the health field are usually indicated by an acronym which relates to certain identifying characteristics of its location, symptoms or consequences.

There have previously been several outbreaks of the coronavirus strain, as in the case of SARS-CoV which emerged in China in 2002 and whose acronym corresponds to Severe Acute Respiratory Syndrome, referring to its symptomology. The MERS-CoV virus emerged in Saudi Arabia in 2012 and its initials refer to the Middle East Respiratory Syndrome Coronavirus, describing both its location and symptoms. The acronym for COVID-19, which emerged in China in 2019, refers to the Coronavirus disease of 2019, with no indication as to its symptoms or source.

It should be noted that COVID-19 was not the first name to be used in the identification of this disease, but it was a term introduced almost two months after the first case was reported to the WHO. This has led some to argue that the motivations for changing and assigning it an 'official' name, were done to avoid the negative consequences of associating a type of disease with a region or population (@radioskyl,2020) (See Illustration 8).

The aim here would be to eliminate the names of 'China virus' or 'Wuhan virus', terms which point directly to the source of the infection. Some health professionals denounce this deference towards China, since the same consideration has not been shown towards other populations, as in the case of the Middle East Respiratory Syndrome Coronavirus, for instance.

As demonstrated in the previous section, despite the fact that an official name of COVID-19 has been assigned, the population has continued to use the terms 'virus' and more primarily 'Coronavirus' to find out about the symptoms, prevention measures and extent of this disease, and although it is still too early to understand the reason as to why the official name has 'failed', it must be taken into account that to create a new brand that is adhered to, a number of variables need to be taken into account, as analysed by Taylor's University in Malaysia (Pool, 2016).

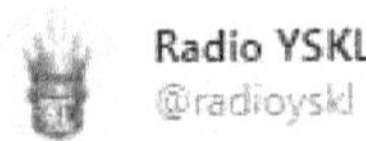

El director de la Organización Mundial de la Salud (OMS), Tedros Adhanom Ghebreyesus, anunció que se cambió el nombre del coronavirus a "COVID-19". Una abreviación de la enfermedad que causó la muerte de más de 1.000 personas.
La primera vacuna "podría estar lista en 18 meses".

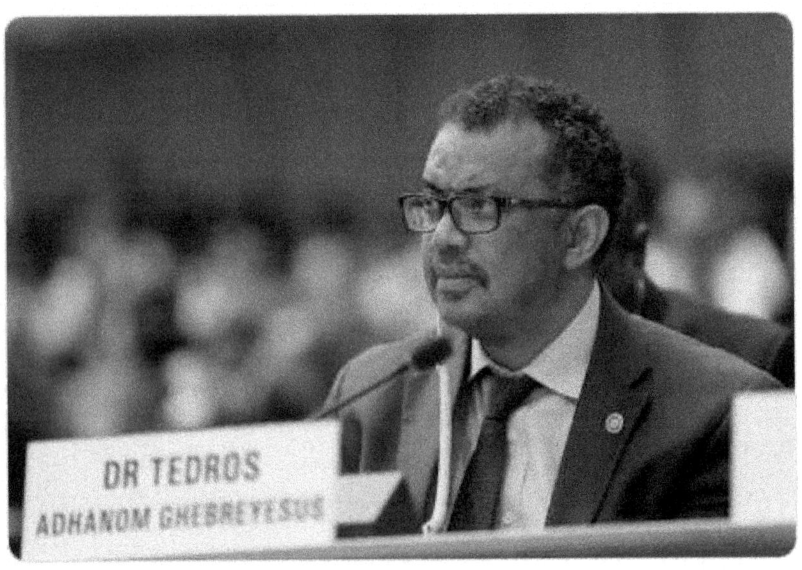

7:22 p. m. · 11 feb. 2020 · Twitter Web App

Illustration 8. Tweet - Name of Covid-19

[Director-General of WHO, Tedros Adhanom Ghebreyesus announced that the name of coronavirus has changed to COVID-19. An abbreviation of the disease that has caused the death of more than 1,000 people. The first vaccination "could be ready in 18 months"].

This research aimed to uncover the reasons for the success of certain brands versus the rest. To this end, a selection of fifty best-selling everyday products from the two main marketing companies was chosen in order to verify the brand's effectiveness. After analysing the messages, pamphlets and publicity of the two brands circulated by the press and media networks, it was discovered, via the application of textual analysis and the interpretative method of research, that in order to maintain the loyalty of their customers, these brands underpin their foundations upon two principles The first principle is the ability to generate positive emotions, and the second the aesthetics of honesty, that is, that the product serves the purpose for which it is designed, whilst maintaining the advertised quality standards.

It should be mentioned at this point that the WHO, together with UNICEF, are the highest valued international agencies worldwide, according to the WIN/Gallup International Survey (WHO, 2014) which indicated that 72% of those interviewed had a positive opinion of these agencies. It would therefore have been expected that, by now, the search term 'COVID-19' would have been widely adopted. However, it must be taken into account that the announcement of the new name took place on 11th February (see Illustration 8) , whilst worldwide concern began almost a month earlier, on 20th January.

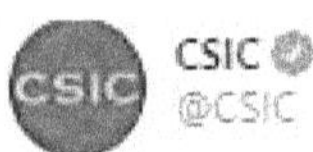

CSIC
@CSIC

El nuevo #coronavirus se llama SARS-CoV-2 y la enfermedad que causa es la COVID-19 (Coronavirus Disease 2019).

En la imagen, virus de la familia Coronaviridae, a la que pertenece el nuevo coronavirus. (Foto tomada por el virólogo Luis Enjuanes (@CNB_CSIC)

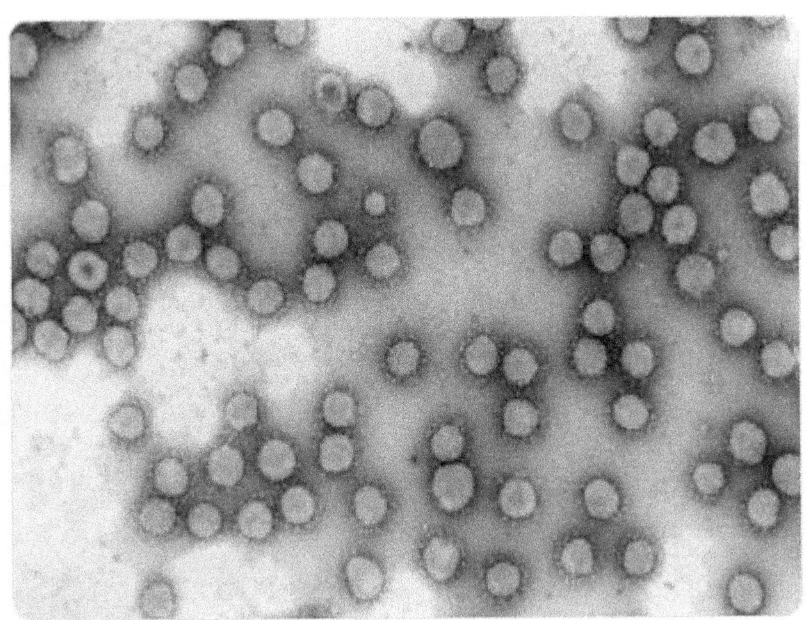

10:45 p. m. · 6 mar. 2020 · Twitter Web App

Illustration 9. Tweet - Image of COVID-19

[The new coronavirus is called SARS-CoV-2 and the disease it causes is COVID-19 (Coronavirus Disease 2019)

There thus remains a tendency for the terms 'virus' or 'Coronavirus' to continue to be used (CSIC,2020) (See Illustration 9).

In the photo, virus of the family Coronaviridae, to which the new coronavirus belongs. (Photo taken by virologist Luis Enjanes (@CNB_CSIC)]

Adoption of Health Measures

One of the most difficult phenomena for people to face is in terms of the adoption of healthy behaviour, which requires some time to accept, understand and assume.

Unlike other phenomena such as the latest trends, which have the ability to motivate the population, when it comes to health, the authorities are often faced with minimal success in their awareness campaigns. Such campaigns aimed at the recommendation of the adoption of healthy habits and behaviour are usually accompanied by restrictions and even penalties for those who do not comply.

However, the population struggles to see any 'benefits' in the short term, resulting in a reduction in any 'interest' and motivation for the adoption of these new habits, to the extent they may not even carry them out at all, thus failing to comply with the authorities' recommendations.

Whilst health is an aspect of concern to society, the concept of prevention is not always understood and accepted in the same way, especially when it comes to the adoption of some behaviours which tend to go against those which are customary (MinInteriorAR, 2020) (See Illustration 10).

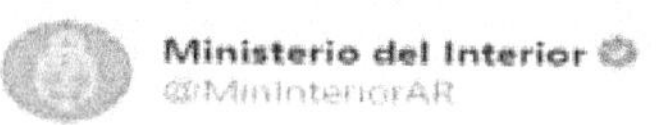

Cuidá tu salud y la de tu familia. Recordá siempre no compartir el mate, la vajilla y demás objetos de uso personal.
Conocé más en bit.ly/Coronavirus-Co...

#ArgentinaUnida #CuidarteEsCuidarnos

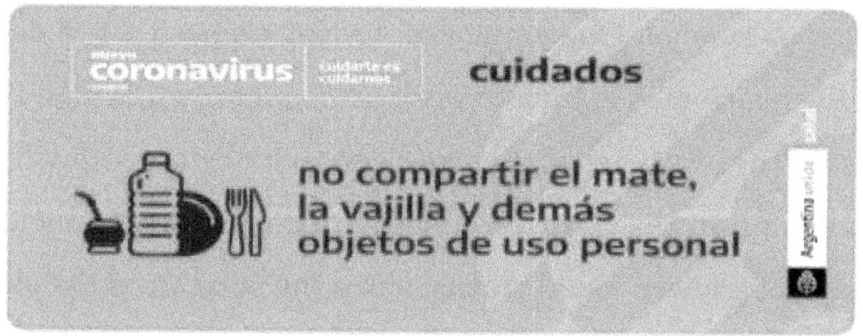

1:00 p. m. · 28 mar. 2020 · TweetDeck

Illustration 10. Tweet - Prohibited Activities

[Look after your health and your family's. Always remember not to share your *mate* [1], your utensils and other personal objects. Learn more at bit.ly/Coronavirus-Co [N]

In the case of COVID-19, the population has been asked to 'abandon' some practices and adopt new ones. Going against 'routine', has made it difficult for many at first to adopt these recommended measures. This is because, sometimes, despite medical guidelines, the population does not acknowledge the risks to their health

[1] Mate is a traditional South American caffeine-rich infused drink.

of certain behaviours, as previously mentioned. One such instance is in the practice of artificial tanning with UVA rays, an activity that has greatly increased in certain countries over recent years.

In some places being tanned has become something of a status symbol. One employee, having enjoyed a few days at the beach may return to work nice and brown, whilst the rest of the office, who have not been so lucky are still white and pale. On the contrary, in other places, being tanned is a sign of a lower social status, since the sun burns the skin of outside workers, giving it that characteristic brown colour, whilst other less manual jobs do not leave that 'imprint' on the body. It can therefore become a signal as to the economic status of the consumer, differentiating between those who can afford it and those who can't.

In Western society today the first approach dominates, that is people feel good about themselves when tanned, something which takes time and in some cases money, to achieve. To meet this demand, a number of establishments have emerged, with UVA lamps which produce the same effect on the skin after one or more exposure sessions. And so, with this UVA ray system, the same tanned appearance is achieved as if one had gone on a relaxing beach holiday in the sun.

So, simply by spending a few minutes inside one of

these devices, one can enjoy the 'benefits' of being considered of a higher economic status.

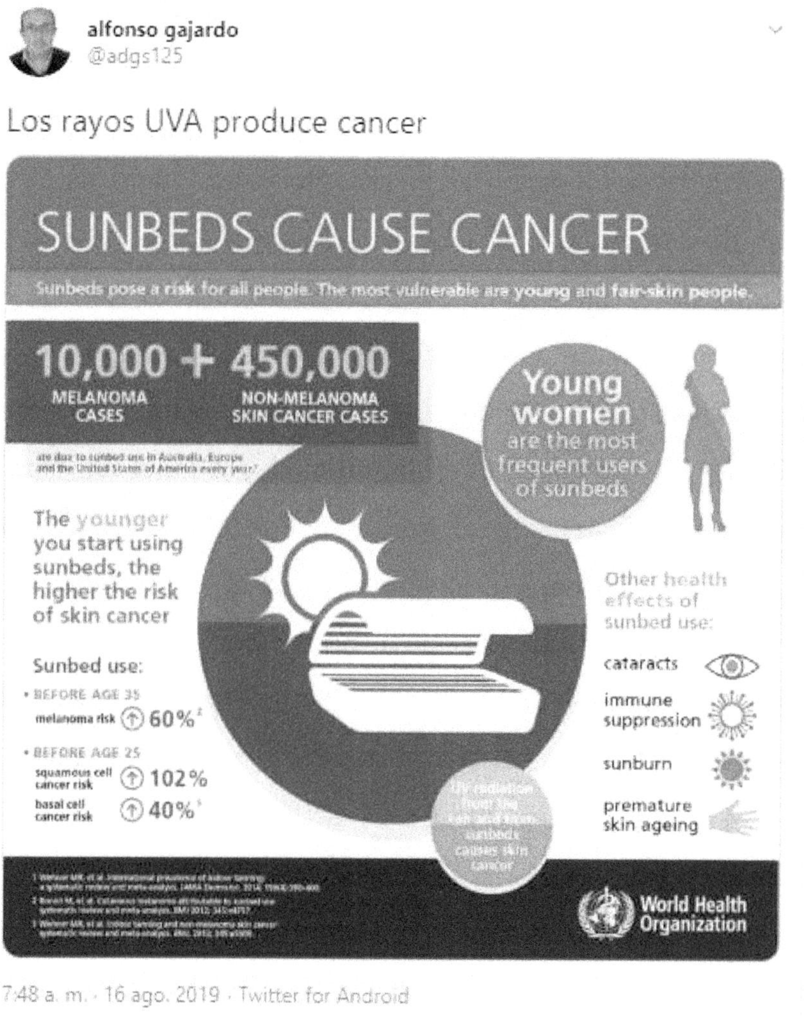

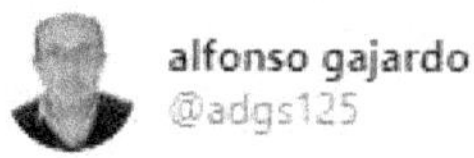

alfonso gajardo
@adgs125

Los rayos UVA produce cancer

SUNBEDS CAUSE CANCER

Sunbeds pose a risk for all people. The most vulnerable are young and fair-skin people.

10,000 + 450,000
MELANOMA CASES
NON-MELANOMA SKIN CANCER CASES

Young women are the most frequent users of sunbeds

The younger you start using sunbeds, the higher the risk of skin cancer

Sunbed use:
• BEFORE AGE 35
melanoma risk 60%
• BEFORE AGE 25
squamous cell cancer risk 102%
basal cell cancer risk 40%

Other health effects of sunbed use:
cataracts
immune suppression
sunburn
premature skin ageing

World Health Organization

7:48 a. m. · 16 ago. 2019 · Twitter for Android

Illustration 11. Tweet - Relation between UVA rays and cancer.

[UVA rays cause cancer]

Despite the popularity of this system, in recent years medical research has been compiled which has discovered associations between the excessive use of UVA rays and skin cancer. Therefore, people who use and, more importantly, abuse these tanning sessions are voluntarily putting themselves at risk to skin diseases (adgs125, 2019) (See Illustration 11).

An investigation has been carried out to assess the psychological impacts of the usage of UVA rays by the Department of Dermatology, Warren Alpert Medical School; Department of Epidemiology, School of Public Health; Medical Centre, Providence VA Medical Centre; and the Department of Psychiatry and Human Behaviour, Warren Alpert Medical School, Brown University; together with Division of Network Medicine, Brigham Hospital; Department of Nutrition and Department of Epidemiology, Harvard School of Public Health; together with the Division of Adolescent Medicine, Boston Children's Hospital; Department of Dermatology, Rhode Island Hospital (EE.UU.) together with the Department of Occupational and Environmental Health Sciences, Faculty of Public Health, University of Peking (China) (Li et al., 2017).

The study involved 67,910 women between the ages of 25 and 35 who were asked regards the frequency with which they used UVA ray tanning rooms. The aim of the study was to determine if there was an association between frequent indoor tanning and other mental disorders such as food addiction. To this end the Yale Food Addiction Scale was used (Flint et al, 2014). The participants' clinical history as to whether or not they had suffered from depression was also taken into account.

The results showed a significant relationship between the presence of depression and greater use of UV rays. Also demonstrated was a significant relationship between the abuse of UV rays and symptoms associated with eating disorders, particularly anorexia.

As with other activities, the use of this type of service may be considered normal, except when control is lost and it becomes an addiction, that is to say it is being undertaken for its own sake, rather than for the benefits it may bring. Such behavioural addiction to tanning is called tanorexia. In this instance, the depressive symptoms appear to play a fundamental role in the formation or maintenance of the addiction to UVA rays, as if the individual attempts to 'offset' their state of mind by giving a 'better' image of themself to others.

Previous research has reported significant relationships between food disorders and depressive symptoms, but in this instance the relationship is mediated by an addictive behaviour, such is the abuse of UVA rays.

According to the conclusions of the study, consideration must be taken with individuals who abuse the use of UVA rays, since it may constitute depressive symptomatology and the suffering of anorexia.

Despite these findings, and the health problems associated with skin cancer discussed earlier, people find it difficult to give up this type of habit, since the short-term benefits of a tanned skin mean any long-term health damage is underestimated.

This type of attitude may also be witnessed in the undertaking of other unhealthy habits or those that entail long-term damage, where the consumer 'assumes' the risk, focussing on the short-term benefits, despite warnings from the authorities. For instance, for some years governments around the world have been trying to stop tobacco use. Furthermore, the authorities have had to 'fight' against the portrayal of this habit in films and the media where, in recent decades it was seen as socially accepted, despite the harmful effects on the health of the consumer and the people around them, in what is known as passive smoking (@CNPT_E, 2017) (See Illustration 12).

Existing measures tend to act in a dissuasive manner by putting all kinds of obstacles in the way of its consumption, stopping short of prohibition. Its display is limited to certain specially designed areas, the price is increased, and images are included on the packs of the negative health effects. However, some governments have decided to take a step further and employ the same mechanisms that for years served to spread and encourage tobacco use - television advertising. But are anti-tobacco advertisements effective?

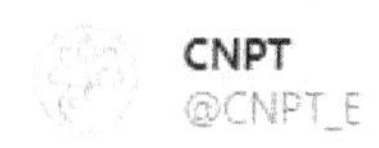

CNPT
@CNPT_E

El #EmpaquetadoNeutro elimina la publicidad del tabaco y ayudaria a reducir la prevalencia del tabaquismo en España cnpt.es/documentacion/...

http://cnpt.es/documentacion/publicac

DOCE RAZONES PARA APOYAR EL EM...
DEL TABACO EN ESPAÑA

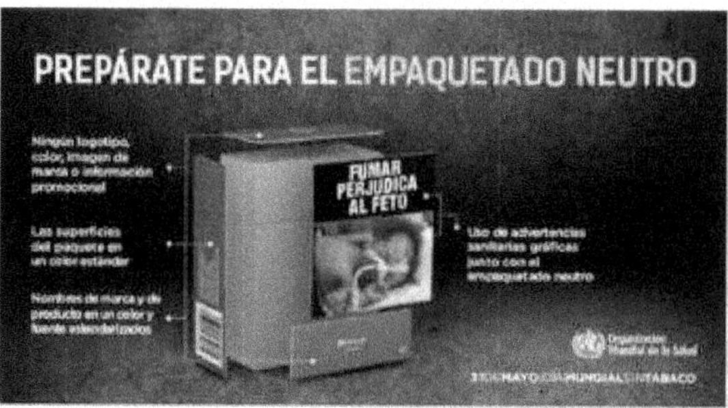

12:39 p. m. · 12 jul. 2017 · Twitter Web Client

Illustration 12. Tweet – Prohibition of Tobacco Advertising.

[The #EmpaquetadoNeutro removes the advertising from tobacco and helps to reduce the prevalence of smoking in Spain]

This question has been addressed in research undertaken by the Department of Education, Seoul National University and the TESOL Department, Hankuk University of Foreign Studies (South Korea); along with the College of Nursing and Health Innovation, Arizona State University and the Department of Psychology, Jesuit University of Wheeling (USA) (Wilson et al., 2017).

The study involved 58 university students who were split into two groups, the first group viewed two emotionally focussed anti-smoking advertisements, whilst the other group viewed two logical, non- emotional type anti- smoking advertisements. Before and after the viewings all the participants undertook three tests, one related to transformation processes, one to depressive symptoms, and the third regards self-esteem. The results showed no significant differences pre or post viewing, either for the emotional or logical advertising, in any of the variables evaluated, i.e. participants appeared to pay no attention to the information given to them about the harmful effects of tobacco usage.

One of the limitations of the study is in the selection of

the population chosen. Undoubtably the advertising is aimed at preventing young people from starting tobacco consumption, but since in many countries young people start smoking from the age of fourteen, a selection of participants from that age group should have been chosen instead of university students.

Despite the above, it should be noted that the effects of advertising are mainly based on repetition of relevant advertisements, to the extent that the information is learned. Therefore, the fact that the advertisements were viewed only once would explain the insufficient effects upon behaviour towards smoking, self-esteem or depressive symptoms.

In the specific case of COVID-19, and to the surprise of some, an unprecedented measure has been adopted, in the prohibition of all advertising regarding gambling. The idea is to prevent people who are spending a lot of time confined to their homes, becoming 'hooked' on gambling, which can lead not only to addiction, but also to economic ruin when monetary gambling is involved.

Considering that there are other concerns in a time of health crisis, people may not consider the adoption of such measures to be a priority. However, the government has primarily undertaken them to prevent the negative economic consequences gambling can bring about, not only in the altering of people's moods which can lead to major depressive disorder, but also economic ruin which may lead to suicide.

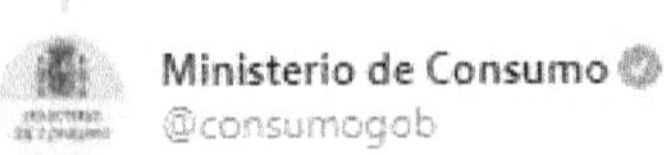

El ministro de Consumo, @agarzon:

"En materia de juego hemos detectado que había un creciente consumo de juego de apuestas online. Por eso hemos prohibido la publicidad del juego en cualquier soporte publicitario, con una excepción en la franja de 1 a 5 de la madrugada."

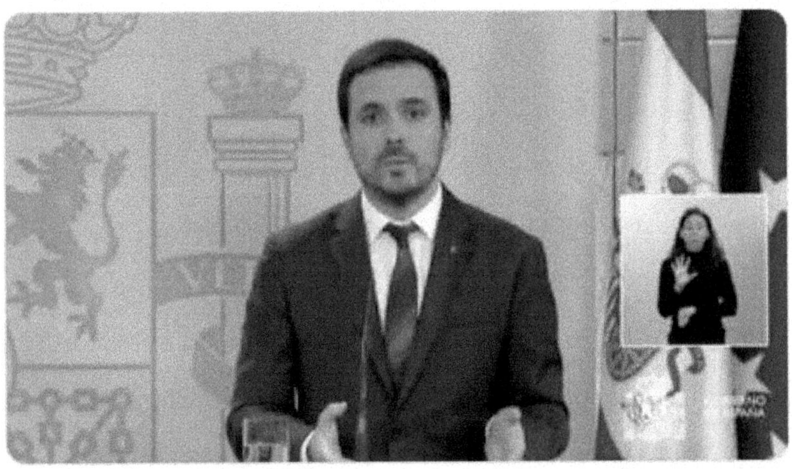

2:31 p. m. · 1 abr. 2020 · Twitter Web App

<u>Illustration 13. Tweet – Prohibition of Gambling Advertising</u>

[Minister for Consumer Affairs, @garzon "With regards gambling we have detected that there has been a growing incidence of online betting. That is why we have prohibited the advertising of gambling in any medium, except during the hours of 1am to 5am."]

Such is the importance in the early prevention of behavioural addictions, for, as time passes, it becomes even harder to 'kick the habit', and in this particular instance, the new addict would continue to play after lockdown. It is consequently important that such measures are adopted in order to prevent negative effects on the physical and mental health of these potential gamblers (-consummogob,2020) (See Illustration 13).

Although such measures might be thought of as exaggerated or out of place, the reality is that our economic behaviour is governed by a multitude of internal and external variables. For example, one usually thinks about shopping in terms of prices. But how much are people willing to spend to buy things? This and other similar questions are dealt with by Consumer Psychology, a branch of study which analyses the behaviour of the individual when faced with varyingly complex economic decisions. The prototype for such investigations concern games of chance, that is, a situation where money may be won or lost dependent upon probabilities that the researcher manipulates.

It has been demonstrated that there are some people

who are conservative in their value judgements, whilst others take more risks. It has also been observed that these personal variables are modified when subjected to temporary or continued consumption of certain addictive substances.

Based on this type of research, other variables, which may be implicated in whether an individual might assume lesser or greater economic costs are analysed, such as obesity. But are there differences in what an individual is willing to pay based on whether or not they are overweight? An answer to this has been sought by research undertaken by the Agricultural and Food Economics Unit, Agricultural Research and Technology Centre of Aragon, Agro-Food Institute of Aragon, University of Zaragoza (Spain), together with the Economic, Agricultural and Food Resources Area, Michigan State University (USA) (De-Magistris, López-Galán, & Caputo, 2016).

The study involved 309 participants, graded as to whether or not they were overweight (those with a body mass index greater than 30 (weight in kilograms divided by height squared) were overweight), and whether or not they accepted their own image in the mirror (using the standardised Body Image State Scale questionnaire (Cash, Fleming, Alindogan, Steadman, & Whitehead, 2002). Four groups were formed, not overweight with acceptance of mirror image; not overweight with non-acceptance of mirror image; overweight with acceptance of mirror image, and overweight with non-acceptance of mirror image.

The study entailed the participants being shown normal or healthy potato crisps, and they had to indicate what price they would be willing to pay for them, with a choice of four pre-set prices.

The results showed that the overweight participants with non-acceptance of their mirror image were those willing to pay the maximum price for a bag of healthy potato crisps, indicating that a willingness to pay for something does not depend solely on price. On the contrary, and as may be understood by the law of supply and demand, other variables such as physiological (overweight) and psychological (personal image) must be taken into account.

Based on these results, in times of lockdown, a gambler may not think of the money they are spending in a logical or reasonable manner, governed by their income and expenditure, but they might well exhibit exorbitant spending behaviour without thinking of any future consequences, thus possibly leading to economic ruin.

For this reason, the aforementioned measures have been very well received amongst anti-gambling associations.

Whilst the measures adopted via the immediate ban on advertising might not appear to be the best way in which to 'educate' the public, experience with other types of health interventions have demonstrated that, despite the greatest of invested efforts, changes are often very slow to take effect.

For example, there remains today much to be done towards the eradication of obesity throughout the world. (@ONU_es, 2019) (See Illustration 14).

This is a public health problem increasingly affecting more countries, whether they are in the 'first world' or those still developing.

This tends to invalidate the explanatory theories for such obesity (appearing at increasingly younger ages) as due to the superabundance and ease of access to food. Social theories are currently being considered to explain how populations with limited food resources, such as developing countries, suffer these same obesity rates (amongst both adults and children).

Although its effects are not as obvious as other public health problems such as smoking or alcoholism, it has many consequences, particularly upon the quality of life of the patient, whose physical activity gradually becomes limited, due to the accumulation of body fat.

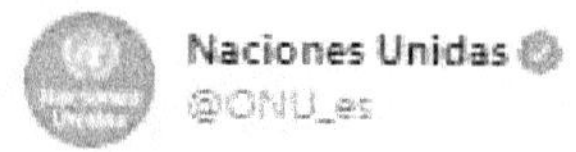

La obesidad es uno de los principales desencadenantes de la diabetes.

América tiene más del doble de adultos con sobrepeso que el promedio mundial. Aprende más sobre los factores de riesgo en este #DíaMundialDeLaDiabetes : paho.org/hq/index.php?o...

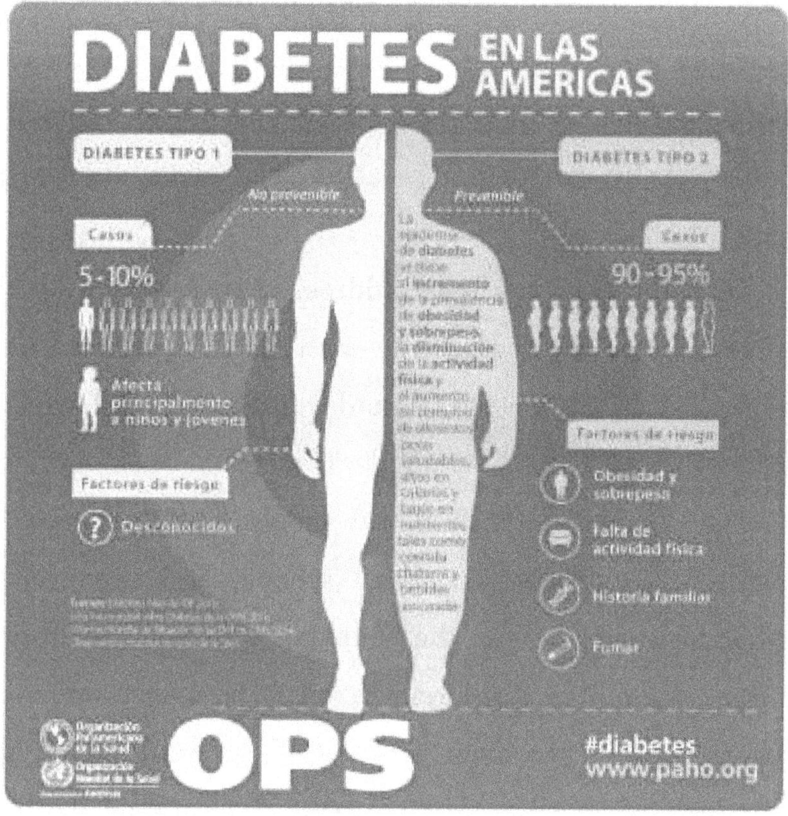

11:01 a. m. · 14 nov. 2019 · TweetDeck

Illustration 14. Tweet- Consequences of Obesity

[Obesity is one of the main triggers for diabetes. USA has

more than double the number of overweight adults than the world average. Learn more about the risk factors here #DíaMundialDeLaDiabetespaho.org/hq/index.php?o..

To combat this problem, efforts have been made in 'educating' from infancy, so children learn to eat a healthy diet. At the same time, in a supplementary manner, many secondary schools and universities provide specific training regarding good nutrition, highlighting the disorders that may arise, such as anorexia or obesity, amongst others. But should health programmes associated with obesity be customised?

This question has been addressed in research by the University of Calgary together with the Health Services of the University of Alberta (Canada) (Russell-Mayhew et al, 2016).

The study analysed 67 awareness programmes on nutrition taught in secondary schools and universities distributed throughout the country. The content of each course was analysed in order to verify how each one dealt with the specific problem of obesity. The results showed a total lack of coordination between the courses, both in terms of the topic and how it was approached, in such a way that only 30% considered obesity as a public health problem. 85% of the courses were oriented to nursing issues in the field of work performance, whilst only 15% of programmes included information on promotion of health via nutrition and adequate exercise. Few programmes emphasised the social and discrimination problems faced by obese patients.

It must be borne in mind that awareness-raising amongst the population is the first step towards achieving some kind of social change, but, if the programmes aimed at such work are inadequate, the problem of obesity will be difficult to solve. The same is true in the changing of behavioural habits or to prevent future addictions, where it is important that clear and precise information is given, with special emphasis on the mediating psychological aspects, so the individual understands what is being said is for the benefit of them and their future health.

List of Illustrations

Referenced Tweets

@adgs125. (2019). Alfonso Gajardo en Twitter: “Los rayos UVA produce cancer https://t.co/iI5wbJdMCn” / Twitter. Retrieved April 4, 2020, from https://twitter.com/adgs125/status/1162239591237079041

@CNPT_E. (2017). CNPT en Twitter: “El #EmpaquetadoNeutro elimina la publicidad del tabaco y ayudaria a reducir la prevalencia del tabaquismo en España https://t.co/F3gWsuRIgW https://t.co/CDGucMDvx3” / Twitter. Retrieved April 4, 2020, from https://twitter.com/CNPT_E/status/885086317775925251

@consumogob. (2020). Ministerio de Consumo en Twitter: "?El ministro de Consumo, @agarzon: "En materia de juego hemos detectado que había un creciente consumo de juego de apuestas online. Por eso hemos prohibido la publicidad del juego en cualquier soporte publicitario, con. Retrieved April 4, 2020, from https://twitter.com/consumogob/status/1245327935768313857

@CSIC. (2020). CSIC en Twitter: "El nuevo #coronavirus se llama SARS-CoV-2 y la enfermedad que causa es la COVID-19 (Coronavirus Disease 2019). En la imagen, virus de la familia Coronaviridae, a la que pertenece el nuevo coronavirus. (Foto tomada por el virólogo Luis En. Retrieved April 4, 2020, from https://twitter.com/CSIC/status/1236045267947970561

@MinInteriorAR. (2020). Ministerio del Interior en Twitter: “Cuidá tu salud y la de tu familia. Recordá siempre no compartir el mate, la vajilla y demás objetos de uso personal. Conocé más en https://t.co/EA3CGrbV1U #ArgentinaUnida #CuidarteEsCuidarnos https://t.co/9OefkoFYX7” /.

Retrieved April 4, 2020, from https://twitter.com/MinInteriorAR/status/1243870452457426946

@NTN24ve. (2018). NTN24 Venezuela en Twitter: "Venezuela entra en la lista de países con crisis humanitaria encabezada por África https://t.co/yb0jKBntG6 https://t.co/mExcSuh9W9" / Twitter. Retrieved April 4, 2020, from https://twitter.com/NTN24ve/status/1005581555719237633

@ONU_es. (2019). Naciones Unidas en Twitter: "La obesidad es uno de los principales desencadenantes de la diabetes. América tiene más del doble de adultos con sobrepeso que el promedio mundial. Aprende más sobre los factores de riesgo en este #DíaMundialDeLaDiabetes: htt. Retrieved April 4, 2020, from https://twitter.com/ONU_es/status/1194918142167932928

@radioyskl. (2020). Radio YSKL en Twitter: "El director de la Organización Mundial de la Salud (OMS), Tedros Adhanom Ghebreyesus, anunció que se cambió el nombre del coronavirus a "COVID-19". Una abreviación de la enfermedad que causó la muerte de más de 1.000 personas. La p. Retrieved April 4, 2020, from https://twitter.com/radioyskl/status/1227296755986903040

References

Cash, T. F., Fleming, E. C., Alindogan, J., Steadman, L., & Whitehead, A. (2002). Beyond body image as a trait: The development and validation of the body image states scale. *Eating Disorders*, *10*(2), 103–113. https://doi.org/10.1080/10640260290081678

de-Magistris, T., López-Galán, B., & Caputo, V. (2016). The impact of body image on the WTP values for reduced-fat and low-salt content potato chips among obese and non-obese consumers. *Nutrients*, *8*(12). https://doi.org/10.3390/nu8120830

Flint, A. J., Gearhardt, A. N., Corbin, W. R., Brownell, K. D., Field, A. E., & Rimm, E. B. (2014). Food-addiction scale measurement in 2 cohorts of middle-aged and older women. *American Journal of Clinical Nutrition*, *99*(3), 578–586. https://doi.org/10.3945/ajcn.113.068965

Google Trend. (2020). COVID-19 - Explorar - Google Trends. Retrieved March 7, 2020, from https://trends.google.es/trends/explore?date=today 1-m&geo=ES&q=COVID-19

Johns Hopkins CSSE. (2020). Coronavirus COVID-19 (2019-nCoV). Retrieved March 7, 2020, from https://www.arcgis.com/apps/opsdashboard/index.html#/bda7594740fd40299423467b48e9ecf6

Jung, K., Shavitt, S., Viswanathan, M., & Hilbe, J. M. (2014). Female hurricanes are deadlier than male hurricanes. *Proceedings of the National Academy of Sciences of the United States of America*, *111*(24), 8782–8787. https://doi.org/10.1073/pnas.1402786111

Li, W. Q., McGeary, J. E., Cho, E., Flint, A., Wu, S., Ascherio, A., … Qureshi, A. A. (2017). Indoor tanning bed use and risk of food addiction based on the modified Yale Food Addiction Scale. *Journal of Biomedical Research*, *31*(1), 31–39. https://doi.org/10.7555/JBR.31.20160098

WHO (2020). Coronavirus (COVID-19) events as they happen. Retrieved March 7, 2020, from https://www.who.int/emergencies/diseases/novel-coronavirus-2019/events-as-they-happen

WHO (2014). La OMS y UNICEF son las agencias más

respetadas en el mundo. Retrieved March 20, 2020, from Noticias ONU website: https://news.un.org/es/story/2014/05/1301751

Poon, S. T. F. (2016). Identifying and Comparing Mystery and Honesty as Emotional Branding Values in Brand Personality Design. *International Journal Of Recent Scientific Research*, *7*(3), 9241–9248.

Russell-Mayhew, S., Nutter, S., Alberga, A., Jelinski, S., Ball, G. D. C., Edwards, A., ... Forhan, M. (2016). Environmental Scan of Weight Bias Exposure in Primary Health Care Training Programs. *The Canadian Journal for the Scholarship of Teaching and Learning*, *7*(2). https://doi.org/10.5206/cjsotl-rcacea.2016.2.5

Wilson, A., Kim, W., Raudenbush, B., Kreps, G., Kim, M., & Wilson, A. L. (2017). The Effects Of Emotional Vs. Logical Anti-Smoking Advertisements On Smoking Discouragement, Depression And Self-Esteem. *Asian Journal of Educational Research*, *5*(2). Retrieved from www.multidisciplinaryjournals.com

World Meteorological Organization. (2020). Tropical Cyclone Naming. Retrieved March 7, 2020, from https://public.wmo.int/en/About-us/FAQs/faqs-tropical-cyclones/tropical-cyclone-naming

Chapter 2. Reactions to COVID-19

One of the biggest problems facing the authorities is in how to manage the population, whilst also complying with recommendations and guidelines for the control of the health crisis, with the minimum amount of infections and deaths.

Historically there are countries which have suffered more due to public health problems. In Asian and African countries, for example, there have been several outbreaks of varying severity, so in these countries the population is more aware of the importance of compliance with government measures, and they are better prepared for coping with a disease than those countries who have not suffered a health emergency for a long time. Regarding the measures recommended by the WHO to deal with the spread of COVID-19, a series of suggestions have been made that have been circulated by governments to their citizens as measures to prevent the spread of the virus and thereby try to control the number affected (@minsalud, 2020) (See Illustration 15).

Although these measures are presented as basic and essential, they do not take into account a phenomenon widely recognised as the IKEA effect. This is whereby the consumer feels better and more fulfilled if they carry out certain actions at a medium level of difficulty, e.g. assembling a prefabricated wardrobe, following the included instructions. This phenomenon was discovered in joint research undertaken by Harvard Business School, Yale University and Duke University (Norton, Mochon & Ariely, 2012), in an attempt to analyse why companies like IKEA had been so successful in recent years.

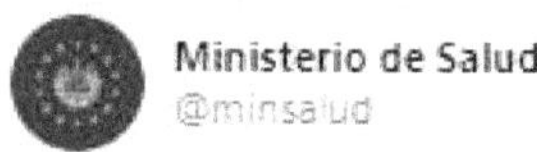

El país se mantiene a cero casos sospechosos y cero casos confirmados de coronavirus (COVID-19).

Unámonos a la prevención de esta enfermedad siguiendo estas recomendaciones:

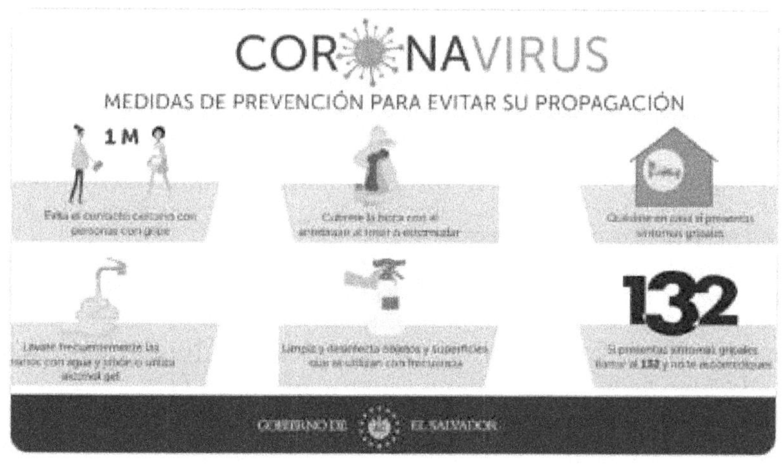

4:32 a. m. · 1 mar. 2020 · Twitter Web App

Illustration 15 Tweet - Measures against COVID-19

After checking a multitude of variables, the researchers realised that a client's involvement in the 'construction' tasks via the assembly of elements according to a predetermined diagram, seems to create a certain degree of personal satisfaction for having completed a creative activity.

In order to prove this, the researchers used various tasks in which volunteers participated. The participants were then asked to financially evaluate the final product for each of the assigned tasks, whether they were those closest to the 'normal' IKEA type of activity, like putting a box together, or others, like making a paper figure using the technique of Origami.

The results reported that, so long as they were permitted to finish, the 'constructors' valued their work more, even when compared alongside work completed by experts, which despite looking better, did not generate the same level of satisfaction. Therefore, constructing something with one's own hands, despite the fact that it may not be properly assembled, increases its subjective value, even when compared to an already assembled item for sale. This has been dubbed the IKEA effect, named after this same company who has popularised 'do it yourself', and it has already been observed in other brands and companies who offer this creative participative experience in the construction of a final product.

Extrapolating these results to the current actions being taken by the population to stop the spread of COVID-19, if these measures should involve a medium level of difficulty, the public will feel satisfied that they are effectively contributing to the spread of disease, however if they are only asked to take low-level measures, such as washing hands or keeping their distance, this will provoke a certain feeling of lack of involvement, since they will feel that 'everything is in the hands of the government' which could lead to a feeling not only of dissatisfaction with the situation, but a lack of adherence to said measures.

In many instances, due to a lack of awareness or foresight on the part of the authorities, psychological aspects may be behind the limited effectiveness of certain campaigns for the adoption of specific health behaviours,. For example, when it comes to lockdown measures which do not involve any 'special' activity, this may lead to the individual feeling a certain sense of disappointment in that they are doing nothing, whilst they see other professionals like health workers and law enforcers often stretched to the limit and beyond in fighting this pandemic. Therefore, when specific initiatives have emerged for people to contribute from home, for example the use of 3D printers in printing equipment for hospitals, or even for making masks, they have taken on the tasks with the feeling that they are actually doing something to combat the negative effects of COVID-19 (Newtral, 2020) (See Illustration 16).

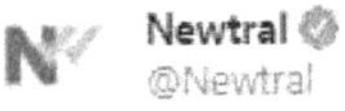

Newtral
@Newtral

Mascarillas, viseras e incluso respiradores. Miles de personas con impresoras 3D están intentando ayudar al personal sanitario creando material EPI en sus casas.

newtral.es/makers-una-imp...

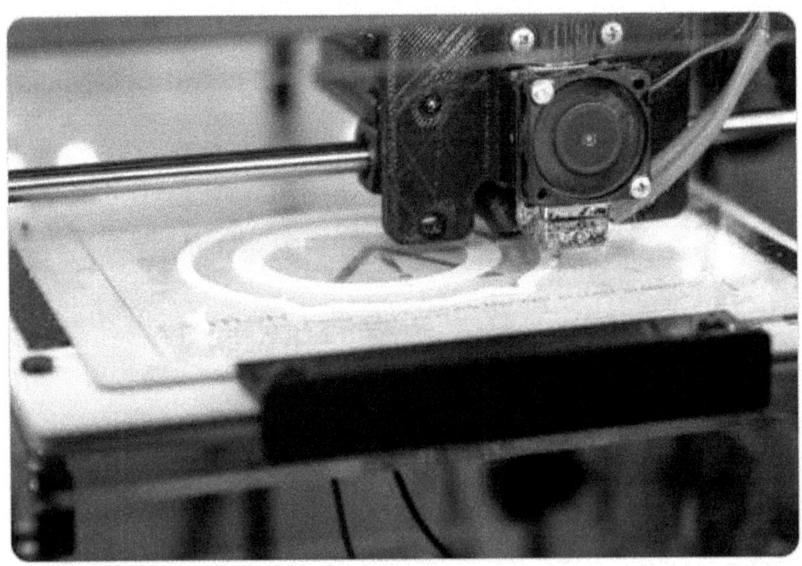

2:24 a. m. · 31 mar. 2020 · Buffer

Illustration 16 Tweet. The Volunteering of 3D Printers

[Masks, visors and even ventilators. Thousands of people with 3D printers are trying to help health personnel by making PPE in their homes.]

Such actions of solidarity have not stopped there, as some altruistic people have volunteered to shop and distribute their purchases amongst the elderly in their homes. This has avoided the necessity for older people to go outside, thus exposing themselves to the virus since, according to some statistics, this is the group which remains the most unprotected against the negative effects of COVID-19.

Although what is currently being experienced is an exceptional situation, every year the population is exposed to the phenomenon of seasonal flu, which has a major effect, especially amongst the most vulnerable groups. And so, with the arrival of the cold season, the media, following the advice of the Ministry of Health, reveal series of recommendations aimed at preventing the spread of the illness, as well as reporting on the advisability of getting vaccinated to avoid it, particularly amongst high risk groups. This is a customary procedure, but something which is backed by a great deal of psychological analysis as to how different groups respond. Hence the campaigns aimed at increasing public awareness of certain healthy behaviours involve both planning and study in the identification of the objective, then getting as close as possible to the target population, who are often the most at-risk groups.

Much progress has been made in the implementation of sales or advertising techniques with regard to 'reaching' the individual, but when it comes to health it is not so easy. Big brands, with repeated advertising exposure can 'make it easier' for us to buy a product or service, but does it work the same way with health?

When health institutions like the WHO or government departments wish to implement a campaign to promote healthy behaviour, whether it be exercise, food or vaccinations, they tend to encounter a major problem - that of the limited effect of their campaigns. Amongst the explanatory theories for this is the 'difficulty' presented by adults in changing their habits and customs, since there is a tendency for people to repeat their learned behaviour, never questioning if it is for the best or not. Thus if, after repeating the same behaviour year after year, someone then tries to change it, there will be a great deal of 'resistance', despite the fact that the recommendation is in the interest of the individual's health. Therefore, in order to solve this problem, the decision is often made to orient such campaigns towards younger people, the desire being for them to be educated in good habits which will then be maintained for the rest of their life (@maestrocarlosef, 2019) (See Illustration 17).

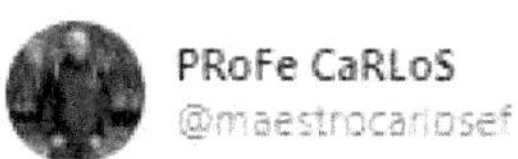

Y llegó el día, hoy 12 de noviembre de 2019 celebramos el Día contra la obesidad infantil desde el proyecto del @CaMiNoPieFCiToS con la campaña DA UN SALTO CONTRA LA OBESIDAD INFANTIL en la que llenaremos los centros educativos de combas sumando SALUD youtu.be/sK3S8VssznI

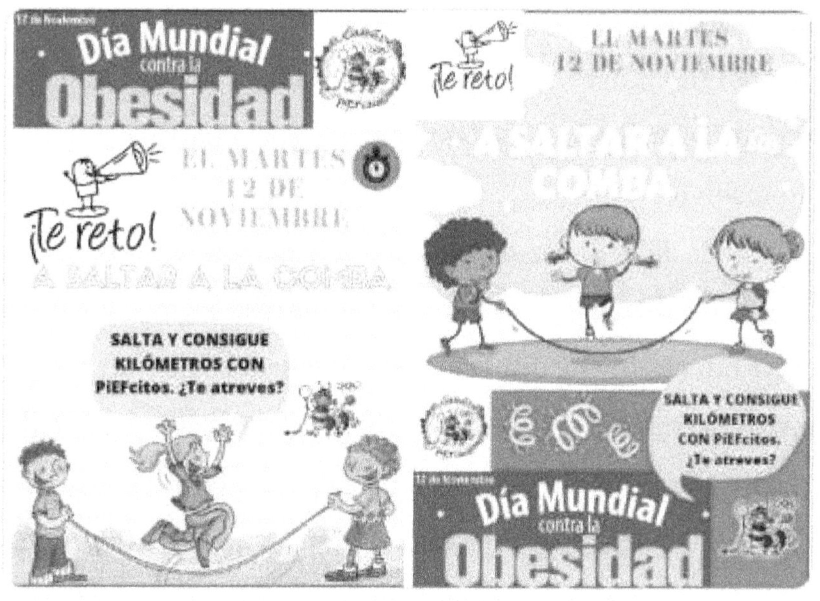

Consejo COLEF y 9 más

5:24 a. m. · 12 nov. 2019 · Twitter Web App

Illustration 17. Tweet - Anti Childhood Obesity Campaign

[The day has arrived. Today, 12th November 2019 we're celebrating Anti Childhood Obesity Day with the project from @CaMiNoPieFCiTos with the campaign TAKE A JUMP FOR THE FIGHT AGAINST CHILDHOOD OBESITY when we will be filling our educational centres with skipping ropes]

The main limitation of this type of intervention is that the long-term benefits cannot be evaluated, because a follow-up of years or even decades would be required to check for changes in the population. Furthermore, these campaigns must fight against all manner of false beliefs or 'gossip' which spreads faster than the health campaigns themselves.

Such is the case with vaccines, which tend to be 'discussed' with a total lack of scientific rigor concerning their effects in the appearance of disorders like autism, for instance, or in the case of the flu vaccine, are considered as 'a thing for the elderly' or 'I had one a year ago so surely I'm still covered'. So how effective are vaccine campaigns?

This question was addressed in studies carried out jointly by the Department of Health and Behavioural Sciences at the University of Denver, Colorado; the Center for Infectious Disease Analysis and Modelling, Yale School of Public Health; the Department of Psychology at Rutgers

University (USA); together with the Department of Epidemiology and Contagious Diseases at the London School of Tropical Medicine and Hygiene (England) (Li, Taylor, Atkins, Chapman, & Galvani, 2016).

The aim of the study was to analyse the effects of a vaccination campaign amongst Internet users, to see if there were any changes in trend.

The study included 4,023 participants over the age of eighteen, from eight countries (Brazil, China, France, Israel, Japan, the USA, UK and South Africa).

Participants were randomly assigned to one of four conditions according to different types of advertising scenarios in which they read a message about flu vaccination, one involved a young victim of flu, one an elderly victim, one with unidentified victims, and one with no message. Three aspects were evaluated – sympathy, general prosociality and vaccination intentions.

Results showed sympathy for all the flu victims, with the young victim eliciting greater sympathy.

With regards prosocial content (measured by the participants' likelihood of donating to an unrelated cause), prosocial motives were stronger amongst historical non-vaccinators, with no difference between young or older participants in this regard. Finally, concerning intention to vaccinate, there were no significant changes in any of the groups, with the biggest predictor being previous vaccination behaviour.

According to the study results, people seem unwilling to change their opinion regarding health issues, therefore work would need to be done via awareness-raising strategies in order to 'educate' the population and counter false beliefs.

Returning to the recommendations concerning COVID-19, there are some measures which are quite basic and easy to carry out, such as repeatedly washing one's hands, or maintaining a distance of one metre from each other. In contrast, other government measures are not so easy for the individual to adopt, as in the case of lockdown, where one is not allowed outside the home without just cause, and to do so risks arrest and prison, or at least a heavy fine.

The practice of lockdown was instigated in China for the first time on 24th January 2020, much to the amazement of the rest of the world.

Millions of citizens were confined to their homes in a move which would previously have been thought impossible due to the number of people involved (@shildalys, 2020) (see Illustration 18).

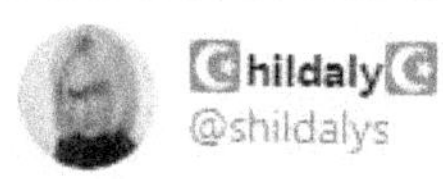

#coronoavirus 24 d enero 2020: #China pone en cuarentena 8 ciudades más en la provincia d Hubei, atrapando a 35 millones de residentes en sus ciudades. Al cierre d esta edición, 2019-nCoV ha matado a 26 pacientes, todos en China. En todo Estados Unidos, 63 casos no confirmados

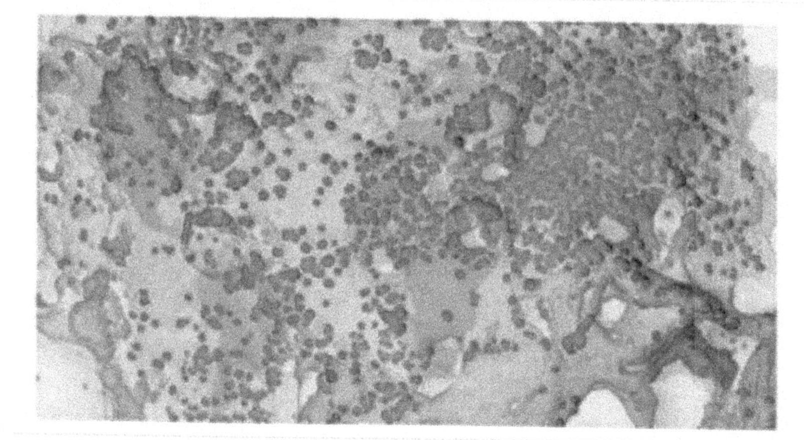

1:35 a. m. · 25 ene. 2020 · Twitter for Android

Illustration 18. Tweet – Lockdown in China

[24th January 2020 #China places 8 more cities in the province of Hubei in lockdown trapping 35 million residents in their cities. At close of this edition 2019-nCoV has killed 26 people, all in China. In all of USA 63 unconfirmed cases.]

This is a controversial decision with regards the limitations it imposes on the individual concerning rights of movement and even work, but a necessary measure in times of a health crisis, in an attempt to halt the spread of disease for the benefit of the community as a whole. This aspect, however is not always understood, and for this reason governments have invested millions in media and social media advertising campaigns to 'change' how this restrictive measure is viewed, that is, as a necessity in the current circumstances.

Following the decision taken by China, and based on the increasing number of detected cases, Italy carried out the same restrictive measures in respect of movement in some of their northern regions. This decision was adopted on 7th March 2020 (See Illustration 7), then increased to cover the whole country. From that time on other countries have been adopting similar methods, from partial or total closure of non-essential activities to literally closing borders to prevent 'infected' foreigners bringing in the disease (@Renzo_Utili, 2020) (See Illustration 19).

Perhaps the most controversial measure in China, apart from lockdown, is the authorities' recommendations to their citizens that when someone has the symptoms of COVID-19 they should go to hospital, furthermore, if they know a family member or even just a neighbour suffering from it, that they tell the health authorities.

Renzo
@Renzo_Utili
ITALIA aisla en rígida Cuarentena a 16 Millones de personas, nadie podrá salir o entrar solo por motivos muy urgentes: mapa
Monza Brianza
Verbano Cusio-Ossola
Como
Sondrio
Lecco
Varese
Bergamo
Treviso
Novara
Brescia
Vercelli
Milano
VENETO
Padova
Venezia
PIEMONTE
Lodi
Cremona
Mantova
Pavia
Piacenza
Asti
Alessandria
Reggio Emilia
Parma
Modena
EMILIA-ROMAGNA
Rimini
Le province in cui si può entrare e uscire solo per gravi motivi: mappa
L'ingresso in Lombardia e in alcune zone di Veneto, Emilia Romagna e Piemonte sarà consentito solo per motivi «gravi e indifferibili». Lo prevede il decreto che ...
corriere.it
12:52 p. m. · 8 mar. 2020 · Twitter for Android

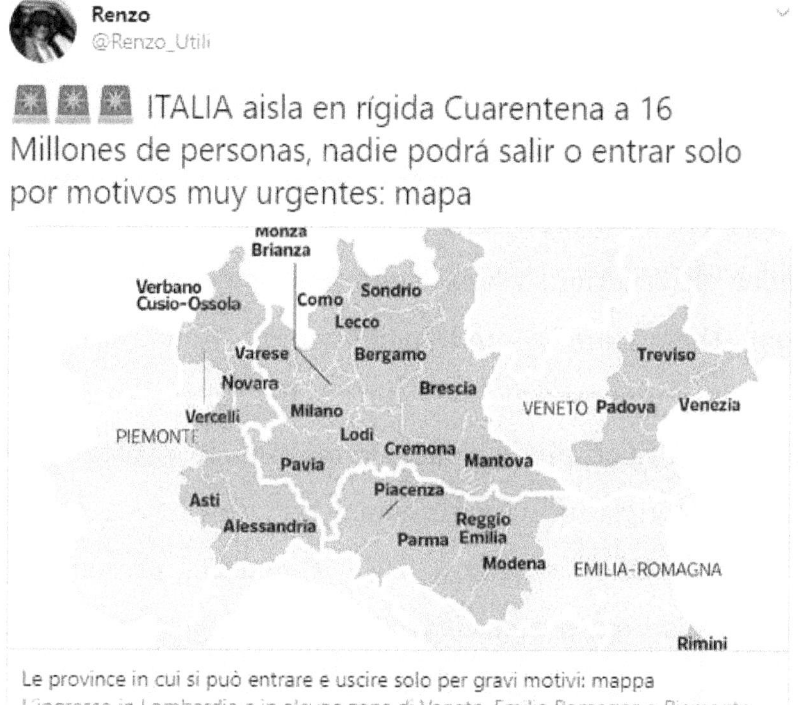

Illustration 19. Tweet- Lockdown in Italy

[Italy imposes strict lockdown on 16 million people, no one can leave or enter except for urgent reasons: map]

Whilst such a health measure is essential for the care of those infected, it may lead to a moral dilemma for the person who must report a possible case to the authorities. On the one hand, the measure means the patient will be treated in a hospital and the virus will not be spread to other people, but on the other that patients may be taken away and not come back.

The reasons for patients not returning home may vary, from death to intensive care hospitalisation. They may even have recovered from the disease but are being kept under observation, which could entail weeks of isolation from their family and neighbours, who receive no information regarding their state of health and recovery or otherwise. Such misinformation may cause a certain level of fear amongst individuals who, when they have a relative or acquaintance with any of the symptoms presented by this disease, are posed with a dilemma as to whether or not to tell the authorities. This causes 'mixed emotions', a phenomenon which social psychologists have sought to explain, long recognised in the story of human nature and closely related to an individual's moral development.

The Northwestern University have analysed the extent of ease with which whistleblowing is carried out in the business field, for what are labelled manifest injustices (Dungan, Young & Waytz, 2019). The study found that a worker's whistleblowing response is based exclusively on their own moral judgement and, more specifically, based on the two concepts of loyalty and fairness. Loyalty, in this context, to the company for which one works and is paid by, and to bosses and colleagues, despite the fact of their committing irregularities. And fairness, in reporting what is inappropriate and morally wrong, regardless of who carries it out or any consequent risks to one's own employment and economic status.

The study reports that people have certain 'moral tendencies' by which they are governed, so that someone who is loyal will never whistleblow, on the other hand an individual governed by fairness will always do so. The study also attempts to verify how 'rigid' moral conventions are. To this end, 293 participants were asked to write a short essay on either fairness or loyalty, dependent upon which group they had each been assigned to, and they later had to resolve a situation in which they had to decide whether or not to whistleblow. The results indicated that the participants who wrote about fairness largely took the decision to whistleblow, whilst for those who had to write about loyalty, almost all of them decided not to.

Despite being an experimental study, the conclusions drawn seem clear, suggesting that morality will play a fundamental role when following current health authority recommendations for the 'reporting' of a relative or neighbour presenting symptoms associated with COVID-19.

It must be borne in mind that every day individuals are

faced with different decisions and they make them in the light of moral concepts internalised during childhood. This morality can change in the light of new experiences, whether direct or indirect, that is to say people learn from experiences observed in others. Futhermore, these experiences will be influenced by the demands of the outside world, in other words the rules of conduct, correct behaviour and established laws, as well as the information and publicity received by the mass media which can 'temporarily' alter our own morality in favour of one behaviour over another. As indicated above, although the moral component does not form part of the personality, it has a similar development, in that the first years of life determine the internalisation of the norms and rules of the society in which one lives. However, unlike personality, morals are more variable, capable of being either flexible or rigid, dependent upon each different experience, and they are also mouldable by external factors, particularly institutions, influential people or the mass media.

The research presented reveals the 'weakness' of our morals when exposed to social demands, and it would thus be expected that the number of 'whistleblowing' incidents regarding family and friends in the current circumstances will be higher than they would be in a non-emergency health situation.

The reporting of citizens was a measure originally adopted by China, however lockdown has now been undertaken by other governments of countries where the virus is active, along with encouragement for people to report those who break the rules (@SeremiSaludRM, 2020) (see Illustration 20).

Seremi de Salud RM
@SeremiSaludRM

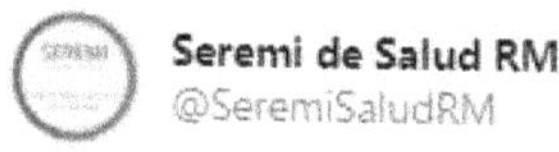

#CuidémonosEntreTodos . Respeta la cuarentena en tu hogar.

Hazlo por ti y tu familia.

Denuncia en

bit.ly/3btyLXE para quienes no lo respeten.

Entre Todos
PLAN DE ACCIÓN
CORONAVIRUS
COVID-19
¡HAZ TU DENUNCIA!
Ingresa a nuestra página web y avísanos si detectas personas incumpliendo su cuarentena o el toque de queda en la Región Metropolitana.
www.intendenciametropolitana.gov.cl

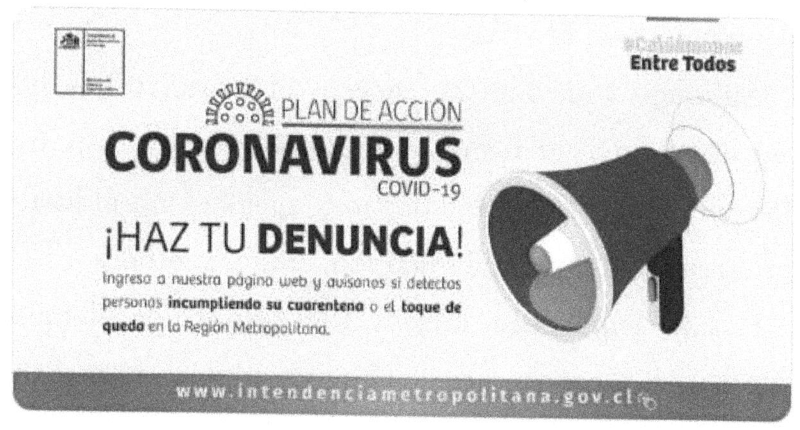

4:54 p. m. · 28 mar. 2020 · TweetDeck

Illustration 20. Tweet- The Reporting of others during Lockdown

[Respect the lockdown measures in your home. Do it for you and your family. Report those who don't comply at. bit.ly/3btyLXE]

In these cases, recommendations by the health authorities are not so much aimed at the reporting of people suspected to be infected with COVID-19, but more concerned with those who do not comply with the lockdown rules, leaving their homes without just cause and thereby exposing themselves to infection, putting both themselves and those they live with at risk. Health workers, law enforcers and other personnel essential for the combat of COVID-19 are exempt from these restrictions, yet they have, on occasions, been rebuked by their own neighbours for putting them at risk.

Although thus far the concept of morality has been used as a univocal term, it is possible to study it from different perspectives, and one may speak of moral justice, moral reasoning or moral emotion, amongst others.

It has long been known that moral development evolves with the maturation of an individual, and that they have more experience with the norms and customs of a specific locality. This is something which is challenged when one goes abroad and encounters 'strange' 'bizarre' or even 'transgressive' forms of behaviour, socially accepted in this particular location, but which would never be permitted in one's own country, and, vice versa, whereby accepted ways of thinking and acting in our society may appear strange and surprising to those from other places.

Many variables have been analysed in relation to morality, as may be seen in the previous study, with the highlighting of the influence of external agents, whether they be institutions or people of influence. But is moral development independent of an individual's intelligence level? This question has been addressed by an investigation undertaken by the Department of Education and Human Development of the Institute of International Education (Germany) (Beiβert & Hasselhorn, 2016).

The study involved 129 minors between the ages of 6 and 8, 52 of whom were girls. For the evaluation of intelligence the Culture Fair Intelligence Test - Scale 1 was used (Weiß, Osterland & Cattell, 1977) while, for the evaluation of moral development, four images representing the transgressing of social norms were presented to the participants, and they were asked how they thought and felt about the scenes. The results did not find any significant differences between the level of intelligence and moral development of the minors, and there was no difference in the data obtained from boys and girls.

As the authors point out, this data contradicts

established theories which mark a parallel performance between operational and moral intelligence based on the theory of moral development (Kohlberg, 1969). According to this theory, in order to have an established morality, a minimum level of personal development, including intelligence, must first be established. However, based on the study data, whether the participants carry out acts of 'whistleblowing' and moral questioning or not will be independent of their level of intelligence.

Decision making is a complex process, as it is not just a matter of choosing between two or more options, but involves a whole cascade of neuropsychological functions.

With regards neuronal-level functioning, outside information first passes through a filtering system in which the limbic system 'gives the go ahead' to such information before an individual becomes aware of it. In this system the amygdala plays a remarkable role in identifying whether incoming stimuli represent any danger or not. If they are of danger, the organism is set in motion in order to be able to give the appropriate 'flight or freeze response' i.e. to either move out of the way of the danger or to stay 'frozen' in the hope that the object of danger does not notice, a remnant from earlier times when our ancestors faced animals which only recognised them as prey when they were moving.

Joy, sadness, anger and guilt are all feelings which 'colour' our way of being and thinking and, ultimately, guide our behaviour. Indeed, advertising specifically seeks to influence the consumer's emotions, by linking them to a particular product or service. When the customer sees the product/service, they remember the emotion the advertisement evoked and they will therefore be more predisposed to purchase it. However, the world of emotions and the influence of the limbic system goes far beyond serving just as a filter or the 'feeling' of positive or negative emotions (Wukmir, 1967), it also plays a fundamental role in attention, learning and decision-making.

Attention is captured immediately by the affectively charged stimuli in front of the 'neutral' ones. Those with a negative charge are attended to earlier and with more intensity, i.e. those which may pose a danger to the individual thus requiring a more immediate response. Once attention has been captured by the affective stimulus, it is easier for the individual to learn or make a decision. It is therefore a basic process, necessary and prior to any other, which occurs in an 'instinctive' way, where the individual has no choice as to what catches their attention or not. Later, once aware of what is happening, they can decide whether or not to pay attention to it.

When one considers learning, it tends to be carried out via 'regulated' studies, i.e. sitting in front of a book and 'swallowing' what is written there. A world away from this type of monotonous and repetitive learning is the kind where we learn 'about everything', not only names, dates and facts (explicit knowledge), but how to do things, like driving, for example, known as implicit knowledge. All learning may either be stimulated within a friendly, pleasant and positive environment, or hindered when these conditions are not met.

Furthermore, any situation that is lived through or recounted to us will be stongly recorded and thus learned, when accompanied by affective stimuli. Everyone can describe a multitude of details surrounding positive events such as a wedding, the birth of a first child....which, despite the passing of time will be remembered as clearly 'as if they happened yesterday'. Similarly, an unpleasant event such as a robbery or a traffic accident and its surrounding details will remain in our memory for a long time. This is why sometimes people find it so difficult to overcome the grief they feel over the loss of a family member or friend, because the vivid memories that they have over such a long period of time cause continued psychological harm.

Having stated the role of emotions in both attention and learning, it should be noted that decision-making, far from being a 'cold and calculated' process, in which the maximum benefit for the individual is sought, it is, in fact, largely influenced by their emotional world.

If we think about the big decisions in our life, who our partner is, what studies we undertake, where we buy a house......we can 'fool ourselves' into thinking we chose it becuase it was the best option at the time. However, if we think it over, we will realise there were a multitude of emotional aspects involved in those decisions, either on our own behalf, or that of other respected individuals who may have advised us. In these times of health crisis, decisions must be made on how best to use available resources and how they should be prioritised. Similarly, decisions are being made to temporarily close companies or postpone indefinitely certain national or international events. One of the first of these decisions to be undertaken, despite the economic and social repercussions it was going to cause, was the cancellation of the Fallas festival in Valencia (@VicentGrimalt, 2020) (See Illustration 21).

This was a very difficult decision for the organisers, who had to choose between holding the customary events, or meeting health recommendations concerning the potential danger for both residents and tourists attending. But what variables come into play in the face of such decisions?

A joint study was undertaken by Cambridge University (UK) and Radboud University (Netherlands) (van den Bos, Jolles & Homberg, 2013) in the form of an exhaustive review of published articles on decision-making. It analyses the different factors which influence decisions, paying particular attention to social influence as a modulator of decision-making.

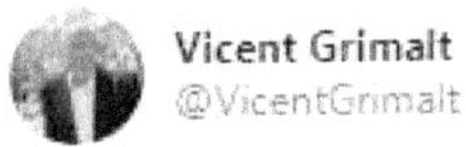

Finalmente, la crisis por el coronavirus nos obliga, por razones obvias de prevención, a aplazar la celebración de las Fallas también en #Dénia, según ha acordado el Govern de la Generalitat.
Entendemos la decepción y la preocupación, pero hoy tocaba tomar esta decisión.

COMUNICADO OFICIAL

La Generalitat, siguiendo la instrucción del Ministerio de Sanidad, ha acordado aplazar la celebración de las fiestas de las Fallas y la Magdalena en la Comunitat Valenciana. La decisión ha sido adoptada por responsabilidad, por indicación de los expertos y pensando en el bien general de la población.

11:05 p. m. · 10 mar. 2020 · Twitter for Android

Illustration 21. Tweet - Cancellation of Las Fallas

[The coronavirus has finally forced us, for obvious preventative measures, to postpone the celebration of Las Fallas also in #Denia as agreed by the Government of Catalonia. We understand the disappointment and concern, but it was the right time to make this decision.]

The learning of behaviour and values via social learning, e.g. group pressure, social comformism, cooperation and social stress, amongst others, are all modulated by the field of emotions.

The study shows that often what weighs most heavily in decision-making, even for those which may have major repercussions for the population, for instance, the establishment of certain government measures, is 'what they will say' i.e. how will the decision be accepted? In the field of politics it often seems that decisions are made to please the electorate or to not lose votes, but in both cases the explanation is the same, the consideration of 'what they will say'.

Whilst decisions made in times of a health crisis are aimed at protecting the health of the population in preventing the spread of the virus, decisions have long been made for altruistic reasons, such as in the case of organ donation, where the death of one person allows another to live. Many health professionals and organisations are trying to raise awareness of the need for donors. The simple gesture of taking out a donor card is all that is required to express the wish of becoming a donor.

Depending upon cultural aspects, there may be a lesser or greater percentage of donors amongst a population, and large differences may be seen between countries in this respect. This indicates that different countries may vary in their awareness of the importance of organ donation, and the positive effects it can have on the lives of prospective recipients who, otherwise, have to continue waiting, knowing that every day spent with a failing organ worsens their quality of life.

The people most willing to become donors tend to be the relatives of organ recipients themselves, since they are more aware of both the need and the usefulness of sharing organs once they no longer of any use to the prospective donor. The testimony of recipients and donors makes it easier for others to become aware of this problem and to become donors themselves, these sentiments can be expressed by the carrying of a donor card.

Despite the above, not all people can be donors, and not all organs given at any one-time may be viable for donation, and health personnel have to make the decision whether the donation may be made or not. However, if an individual does not have a donation card and has not expressed the desire in life to be a donor, it becomes more difficult for health professionals to find healthy organs for donation. Therefore great efforts are made in the media and via talks and awareness days to make people aware of the problem, so they can become donors themselves. But, is it possible to predict if someone will make the decision to become a donor? This question has been addressed by research carried out jointly by the Martin Luther University and the Medicine School Hamburg (Germany) (Hübner, Mohs & Petersen, 2014).

The study recruited 78 university students aged between 19 to 33 years of age, 37 of whom were women. They were all asked about their intention to become organ donors, and their intentions were tested via the Implicit Association Test (Egloff, Schwerdtfeger & Schmukle, 2005; Greenwald, McGhee & Schwartz, 1998) where two stimuli presented on a screen have to be assessed. The study compared the results of explicit responses, that is to say those expressed orally, with implicit responses, those made via a computer. Results showed that the participants who expressed their intention of becoming an organ donor verbally took up more organ donation cards at the end of the study than those who gave implicit responses. Therefore explicitness was a better predictor of behaviour than implicitness in these tests.

These results tend to contradict the usual findings from other areas such as advertising , where participants are interviewed and tested to obtain their opinions regarding a new service or product, and where their responses do not necessarily always correspond to the consequence of purchasing the product.

Perhaps the main difference is that when an individual is faced with these type of decisions, they are not taken lightly but considered in depth so, when asked, their answer is already sufficiently determined, and their decision later demonstrated by the taking out of a donor card. In the study it would be necessary to verify which psychological mechanisms may be involved in a change of opinion, in order to be able to use them in the various awareness-raising campaigns carried out each year, thus increasing their impact by persuading more people to donate their organs at the end of their lives. The decision to give another the chance of better health and a longer life could not be more important. Similarly, in the face of COVID-19, there are decisions which must be taken for the 'greater good', such as those that governments are taking when having to choose between the life and death of certain of their people (@SilenciosaVox, 2020) (See Illustration 22).

With regards to advertising, it should be noted that we are exposed to advertisements on a daily basis, in the press, on the radio, television and the Internet, all of which try to change our way of feeling about a particular product or service. Therefore, when we have to make a choice between several options, we tend to select the one we have heard or seen advertised. This is why advertising companies invest millions to deliver an 'outstanding' advertisement which 'leaves its mark' and, above all, differs from the rest, thus guaranteeing an increase in sales of the product or service advertised.

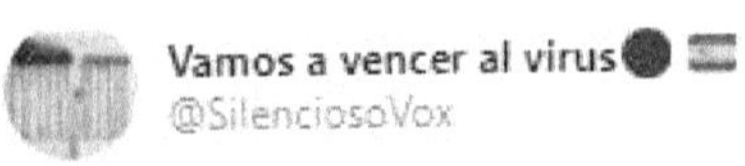

Holanda eres de PM

Países Bajos acusa a España e Italia: "Admiten a personas demasiado viejas con Covid-19 en las UCIs"

El jefe de epidemiología clínica del Centro Médico de la Universidad de Leiden señaló la "posición cultural" que en estos países tienen los ancianos.

8:37 p. m. · 27 mar. 2020 · Twitter for Android

Illustration 22. Tweet – Decisions in the face of COVID-19

[Holland accuses Spain of allowing too many elderly with COVID-19 in Intensive Care Units]

The ultimate goal of these advertisements is to create 'micro emotions' in their viewers, which are significant enough to be remembered when the individual faces a 'real' situation of having to choose between not just the product advertised, but a whole range of alternatives with similar prices and characteristics. The original product is ultimately chosen because a memory is 'stirred' in the individual, from when the advert was first viewed. But how effective are these adverts, broadcast for only a few minutes, yet powerful enough to influence our final purchasing decisions? This question has been addressed by a study undertaken by Tel Hai Academic College (Israel) (Lazar & Pearlman-Avnion, 2014).

The study involved 294 adults, 119 of whom were women. Some of them were presented with auditory stimulation, some negative and some positive which they had to evaluate using the Likert-type scale. Others were given the same task, except the information presented was visual as opposed to auditory. In both groups it was recorded how pleasant or unpleasant the stimuli had been (valence) as well as whether it had caused a lesser or greater emotional impact (arousal). The results reported that, as might be expected, both positive and negative stimuli, whether presented audibly or visually, aroused the expected emotions in the participants. It may therefore be concluded that in decision-making both valence and arousal will play a predominant role, i.e. the product must not only be liked, but liked a great deal, so ultimately that particular product is chosen over others with the same characteristics, offered at similar prices.

Irrational Behaviour

A situation which tends to be feared by most governing authorities is that of uncontrolled mass movements, which can generate chaos and endanger the very survival of society.

Whilst mass movement forms an aspect of sociology, there also exists a fundamental psychological component, the emotions. Emotions are a part of life, whether one is aware of it or not, and are present in every action and decision taken, hence are of major importance to study.

Amongst the theories regarding emotions there are two main trends, those which consider emotions as a univocal and inseparable concept, extending in a continuum from negative to positive affects, and those which consider it as a multidimensional concept, composed of cognitive, behavioural and physiological elements.

Emotion can be considered as a specific 'state' of the individual, allowing him to perceive and respond to the environment (arousal). To simplify, we can consider three possible states, the positive (joy or happiness), the neutral (indifference) and the negative (sadness, unpleasantness, unhappiness). Emotions may therefore be seen as a way of perceiving and responding to the environment, but when this state becomes persistent, it becomes a 'trait' of the personality, i.e. It becomes the individual's usual mode of response to internal or external stimuli.

When persistent emotional states become imbalanced, abnormal emotional processing deviations occur, ranging from the accentuation of anxious or phobic traits, to diseases such as generalised anxiety disorder or major depressive disorder. In addition, it should be taken into account that the environment can impact on emotions, in respect of how one senses and feels, so the more 'critical' the environment, e.g. one that endangers one's life or that of one's loved ones, the more likely it is that the event will emotionally 'scar' the individual. This means that, in the face of a health crisis such as the current one, special care must be taken concerning emotional aspects, in order to avoid instances of confined people suffering some kind of emotional impairment, due to the circumstances in which they are living. Some governments, therefore, make special recommendations in this respect (sanidadgob, 2020b) (See Illustration 23).

Another way of approaching emotion is to consider it as an adaptive procedure of cognitive, physiological and behavioural reaction to environmental or internal stimulation, which may be positive or negative; in other words, emotion affects our body, our thoughts and our behaviour.

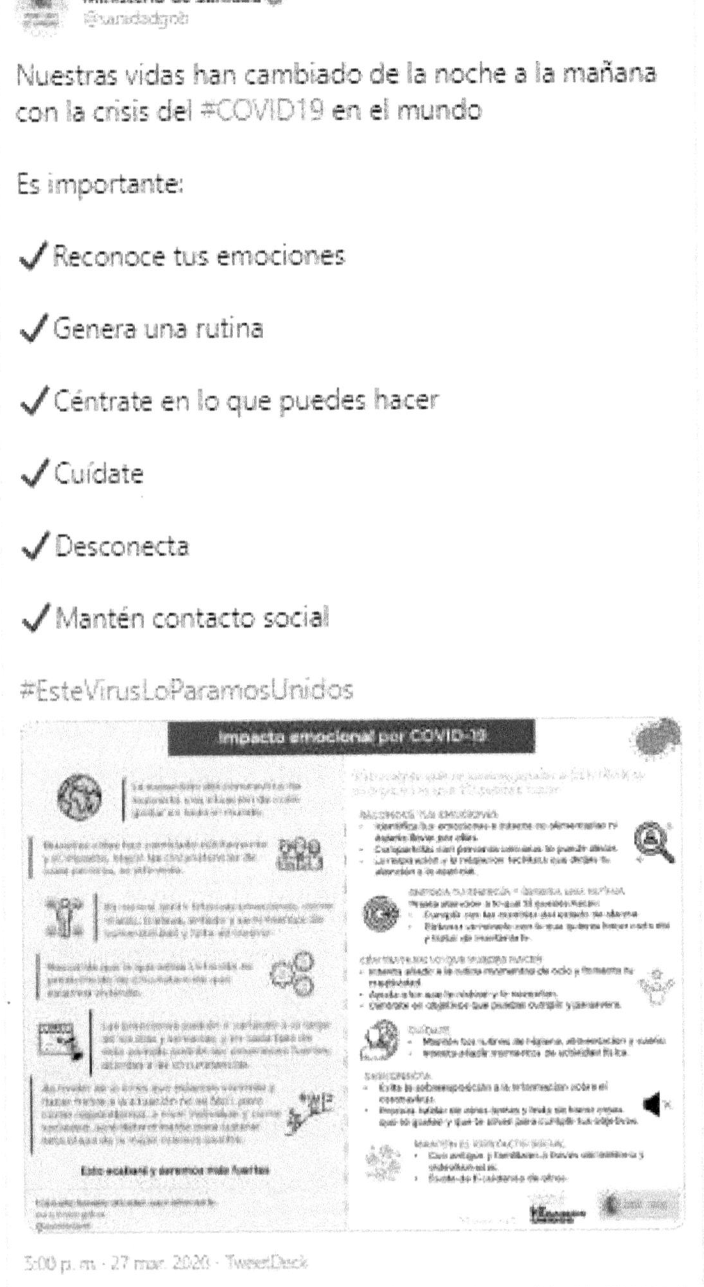

Illustration 23. Tweet – Emotions and COVID-19

[Our lives have changed overnight with the #COVID19 world crisis. It is important to recognise your emotions, keep to a routine, focus on what you can do, look after yourself, switch off, maintain social contact)

Amongst the functions of emotions, the following may be highlighted: coordination of the behavioural response system; modification of the hierarchy of behaviours; provision of communication and social bonding mechanisms; halting or brief retention of cognitive processes; and facilitation of the storage and retrieval of information.

In addition, two more procedures can be identified in the processing of emotion, that of perception and emotional experience. Perception implies a low- level cognitive process, where the emotional stimulus is perceived and evaluated without any awareness or cognitive processing, whereas emotional experience involves high-level cognitive processing, when the perceived is contextualised and interpreted according to previous experiences. A priori these appear to be independent processes, so the processing of emotional perception may or may not involve an emotional experience.

Although up to now affective stimulation has been considered as a unitary concept, emotions may be broken down into three dimensions, that of valence, arousal and dominance (Lang et al., 1997).

The valence dimension refers to the emotional value associated with a stimulus, from pleasant (positive) to unpleasant (negative). This dimension is measured using a Likert-type scale with nine cut-off points from 1 to 9, with value 1 corresponding to the most negative rating, 5 to a neutral rating and 9 to the most positive rating. Measures which positively correlate with this dimension are facial expressions, startle reflex tests, heart rate, and subjective experiences (whether pleasant or unpleasant).

The activation (arousal) dimension refers to the intensity or excitability caused by a stimulus defined as activating (high arousal) or relaxing (low arousal). This dimension is measured on the same scale as above, that is, from 1 to 9, with value 1 corresponding to low arousal, 5 to intermediate arousal and 9 to high arousal. The measures which covariate positively with this dimension are interest level, inspection time, skin conductance, amplitude of P300 component of the Event Related Potentials, and the activation of the occipital cortex using functional magnetic resonance.

The third dimension of dominance relates to the force of submission or dominance caused by the stimulus, a dimension on which there are very few studies.

At the neuronal level, it has been reported that the amygdala plays a fundamental role in the processing of emotions, by influencing cortical areas in three ways (Holland & Gallagher, 1993, 1999): feedback from proprioceptive signals, visceral and hormonal, which allows the body to prepare for action – provoking either the orienting or flight response; projection to networks of general activation or arousal – putting the organism on alert so it can capture threatening stimuli with greater clarity; and interaction with the medial prefrontal cortex – leading to an orientation of attentional resources towards the current emotional stimulus, limiting the rest of the cognitive processes.

For its part, the prefrontal cortex sends different signals to the amygdala, allowing cognitive functions (integrating information from the processing of the emotional stimulus and the context) to regulate the role that the amygdala plays in the processing of emotions. In other words, we respond suddenly (fight or flight response) to the sight of a dangerous animal like a bear (emotional processing), but we do not react in the same manner when that bear is in a cage, within the context of a Sunday afternoon visit to the zoo (cognitive processing).

Emotions are perhaps one of the most studied elements in the field of neuroscience, since one of the differentiating characteristics between humans and animals is the fact that animals are dominated by their instincts and are unable to control or 'cultivate' their emotions. Although, in the first years of life, human 'instinctive' development has been equated with that of other animals, little by little this separates as language emerges and, above, all the control of emotions.

It is currently understood from neuroscience that most decisions made are emotional in nature, and that it is through emotions that one first 'sees the world', and then the decisions made can be rationalised, at least that is how we act when we are faced with different alternatives, of which only one option may be chosen and the rest discarded.

Regarding group behaviour, it has long been known that emotions mobilise people in choosing one direction or another, and in this manner, power groups are able to 'direct' their followers to comply or not with established norms. It is therefore important that political groups and civil and religious institutions maintain the same discourse, one that is not going to 'divide' society in a crisis situation. For, regardless of their own beliefs, designated or 'natural' leaders, with their positive affective responses, are able to mobilise the populace, making the people distrustful of what anyone else may say.

In fact, in the face of the urgent need for information, and the lack of responses from the authorities in some instances, several YouTubers, who previously nobody followed or listened to, have become natural leaders, providing information and explanations in order to satisfy people's curiosity, even though their words do not always conform to the official discourse of the health authorities.

There has, in fact, due to this 'information gap', been an exponential increase in the number of hoaxes surrounding COVID-19, e.g. how it is transmitted and how to 'cure' it, to the extent that the Spanish health service has undertaken an entire campaign against such disinformation (@sanidadgob, 2020a) (See Illustration 24).

However, when it comes to irrational behaviours, these involve a cognitive component, where one acts differently to the expected behaviour within surrounding societal circumstances.

Emotional 'contagion' can occur in crowds, when certain beliefs which generate certain feelings (positive or negative) are spread more or less uncontrollably, being greater in respect of high-activation emotions such as euphoria, anger and rage, which chiefly relate to the primary emotions of joy, anger, fear and sadness.

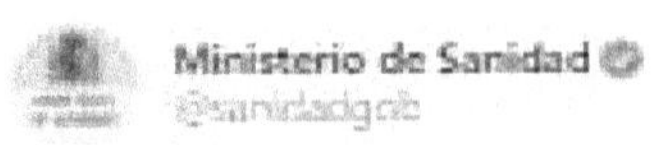

La limpieza adecuada y frecuente de las manos es más eficaz que el uso de guantes, porque:

Usarlos durante mucho tiempo hace que se ensucien y puedan contaminarse

Quitarse los guantes sin contaminarse las manos no es sencillo

#EsteVirusLoParamosUnidos

¿Debo utilizar guantes cuando salgo a la calle para protegerme del coronavirus?
NO, cuando salimos a la calle, la limpieza adecuada y frecuente de manos es más eficaz que el uso de guantes, porque:
LO PARAMOS UNIDOS

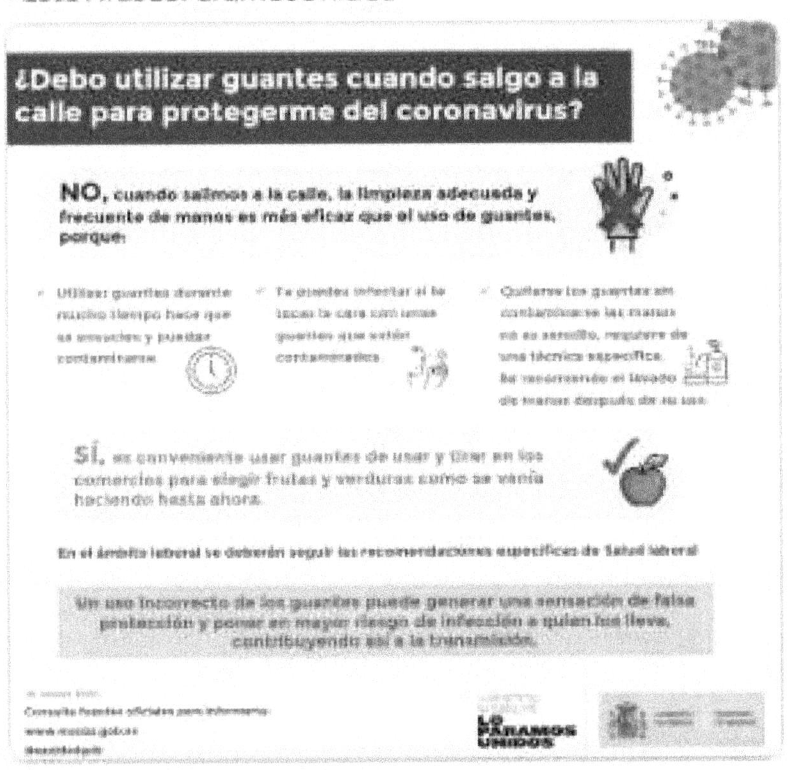

9:56 a. m. · 3 abr. 2020 · Twitter Web App

Illustration 24. Tweet - Information Campaign

[Adequate and frequent handwashing is more efficient than the wearing of gloves because:
Using them for a long time makes them dirty and they can become contaminated.
Taking off your gloves without contaminating your hands isn't easy.]

Social media are playing a decisive role these days in the distribution of certain messages, which are currently being monitored and filtered by large internet companies such as Facebook, Twitter or YouTube, in order to prevent specific messages or images from spreading. This is aimed at the prevention of false news or 'fake news' which has done so much damage in recent years to various societies, since it tends to have an influence on the voting trends of millions of voters. Although it is not a new phenomenon, thanks to social networks a news story can now have a worldwide impact.

Given the capacity of these networks for emotional contagion, the subject matter which is dumped on them is continually being monitored, and images, videos or messages are checked and 'filtered'. Those detected as 'taking advantage' of the situation by promoting primary, mainly negative feelings which are aimed at making a socially difficult situation for the authorities to contend with, are eliminated.

Along the same lines, it can be seen how, even in times of a health crisis, social networks are being used in an attempt to obtain political revenue from both opposing sides, so government supporters will applaud the efforts being made to contain the virus, whilst opponents focus on criticising the harsh measures being adopted.

RSF España
@RSF_ES

COSTA DE MARFIL | Fuertes multas para dos periodistas por publicar "noticias falsas". RSF expresa su preocupación por este paso atrás en un país que llevaba varios años mejorando en libertad de prensa // Inglés, web de @RSF_inter bit.ly/3alk4Qu

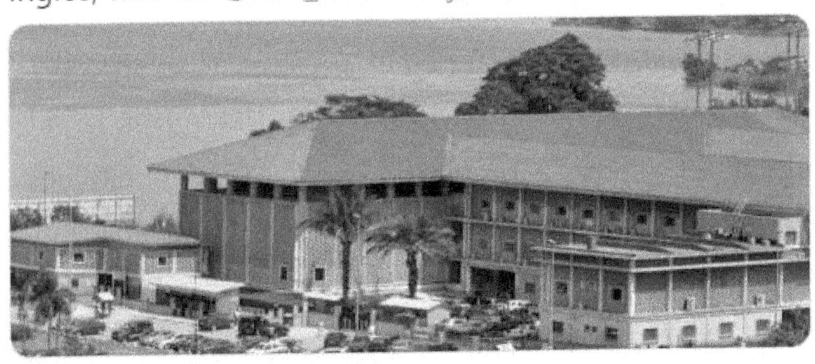

8:16 p. m. · 3 abr. 2020 · Twitter Web App

Illustration 25. Tweet – False Information

[COSTA DEL MARFIL Heavy fines for two journalists for publishing "fake news". RSF expresses its concern about this step backwards in a country that has spent several years improving its freedom of the press.]

And for their part, governments use these same social networks to launch campaigns aimed at reassuring the population, trying to focus on 'positive' instead of negative aspects, and adopting punitive measures against those trying to take advantage of the situation in the way of hoaxes and the spreading of unsubstantiated or patently untrue information (2RSF_ES, 2020) (See Illustration 25).

Racism in the face of COVID-19

Racism is the feeling of identification with a particular race, usually one's own, whilst considering other races 'inferior' or at least 'different'. Historically, racism in some countries has 'justified' many types of violence, underpinned by the sense of belonging to a certain racial group based on the colour of one's skin.

Although racism may be considered 'instinctive' it is, in fact, a cultural and learned aspect of behaviour. This may be demonstrated when one considers places with a multicultural environment and intermingling of races, where little ones grow up considering all races, as well as the mixing of races, as 'normal'. Many countries have had to 'learn' to accept people of other races who, for one reason or another have become just another citizen, and so with time and education should be seen just like any other.

It is consequently the case that populations which are formed mainly from migrants tend to be those most accustomed to a multicultural coexistence. Despite this, amongst their members there are always those who feel that their race or skin colour gives them a kind of 'superior' status to the rest. This is something which is difficult to measure, since in these cultures it is 'frowned upon' to show any feelings of racism, so it tends to be hidden in order to keep up appearances. But can the amygdala expose racism? This question has been addressed by a study undertaken jointly by New York University, the Technological Institute of Massachusetts and Yale University (USA) (Phelps et al., 2000).

In the first study there were 14 participants, half of whom were women, while in the second study there were 13 participants, of whom 6 were women. All participants were white. In the first study they were presented with faces of both white and people of colour with neutral expressions, all unknown to the participants. In the second study faces of well-known people were presented – prominent figures in sports, music or cinema, both black and white. All participants underwent a measurement of neuronal activity via functional magnetic resonance imaging, and the startle response was measured via the evaluation of blinking using electromyography. Furthermore, the participants underwent an implicit attitude assessment procedure using the Implicit Association Test (Egloff et al., 2005, Greenwald et al., 1998).

The results showed an overactivation of the amygdala when the images shown were of people of a different colour to the participant. Such activation was not exhibited when the images shown were of people of the same colour as that of the participant. This does not mean that participants did not react when shown a familiar face or one of their own race, but that the emotional reaction was higher when the image shown was of a person of a different race. Despite the fact that other brain regions were involved in the face-recognition task, only the activation of the amygdala was significant, dependent upon the race of the stimuli presented. Likewise, positive correlations were obtained between the functional magnetic resonance evaluations, the Implicit Association Test and electromyography; therefore, the use of any of the three would be valid for the detection of racism.

There was one surprising outcome concerning positivity with regards the people who were famous in their field, in that a reduction in racism was observed, suggesting that positive experiences, as opposed to none at all, with a particular race, make them appear less different.

It should be noted that, after decades fighting against racism in the USA, a country with a huge immigrant population, the 'unspeakable' sentiment which underpins discriminatory behaviour still persists. For example, although a person may be unaware of it, it is easier for them to help or even hire another of the same race rather than one of a different creed, something which appears quite 'logical' amongst minorities as a way to maintain themselves as a 'people', giving opportunities to 'their own' that, in other circumstances would be difficult. It is, however, detrimental to the concept of integration, because the more a community's sense of group identity is strengthened, the fewer opportunities there are for it to be opened up to new members.

Furthermore, the possibility of knowing that the brain responds to the 'truth', in direct opposition to social conventionalism, facilitates the understanding as to what extent anti-racism campaigns are effective and, if they do not work, how they should be improved, so that gradually this kind of racism can be diluted.

Independent of this racism, which tends to be more or less rooted in society, circumstances may arise which increase a sense of social belonging, marking differences with those who are not the same, or those who, even though they have lived in a particular society for a long time, are singled out and discriminated against due to their skin colour or other characteristic.

Such elements are also used by certain political parties, those based on that particular 'against others' type of identity. They spread nationalist sentiments, such as placing the 'blame' for internal security issues or economic problems on those who do not belong to that society, for instance, on immigrants. Such accusations permeate the thinking of the people who vote for them, thus increasing discriminatory feelings towards the other groups who, in some cases, are the most defenceless.

In other instances, these attitudes may occur due to circumstances unaffiliated with the victimised population, such as in the context of the current health crisis. This disease is known to have originated from a province in China, and there has been an increase in violent acts committed against people with oriental features, regardless of their origins, and also against those who have tried to defend them (-informativost5, 2020) (see Illustration 26).

Behaviour involved in the defence of another person, where one's own personal safety may also be put at risk, demonstrates a high level of altruism and compassion. In a society obsessed with individual outcomes, we sometimes 'turn our back' on the development of compassion, which is seen in many cultures as a 'weakness' in the human being, but, if we stop to think, this is precisely what distinguishes us from animals.

When faced with an old, sick or disabled person, compassion is 'activated' within us and we tend to offer help and protection, something which has also been observed as inherent in our ancestors, since skeletons have been found in graves with healed broken bones, evidence that the group looked after the victim until they recovered.

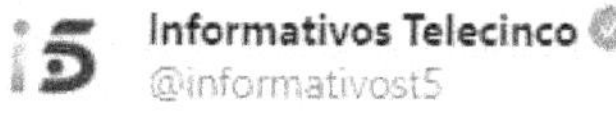

Temor al coronavirus: le propinan un puñetazo por defender a su amiga china

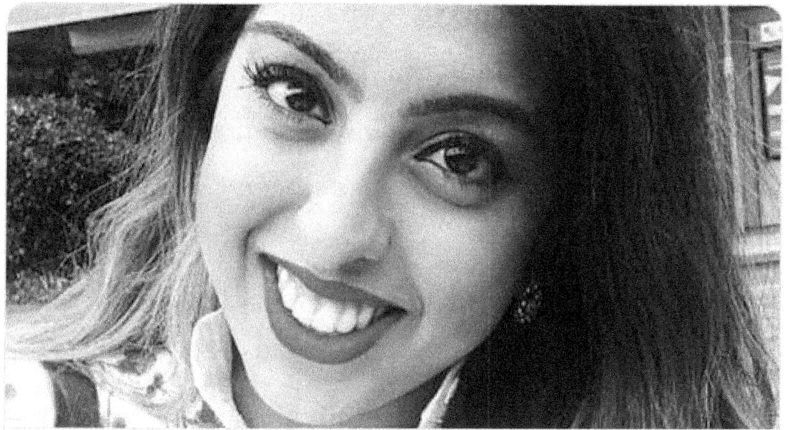

Temor al coronavirus: le propinan un puñetazo por defender a su amiga china
Una mujer ha denunciado la brutal agresión sufrida en una calle de Birmingham, en Reino Unido, tras defender a una amiga suya de nacionalidad...
telecinco.es

2:34 p. m. · 23 feb. 2020 · TweetDeck

Illustration 26. Tweet – Racism during COVID-19
[Fear of the coronavirus: punched for defending her Chinese friend]

People with high levels of compassion tend to get involved with charitable causes, particularly in the event of a social problem or catastrophe, when help is received from real strangers. In addition, compassion may be seen as a protector against negative emotions such as anxiety, anger or fear, fostering instead friendship and social relationships. It is a construct associated with empathy, the ability to understand the emotions of another, thus putting oneself in their situation, but it is equally present in daily life and used to a lesser or greater extent, depending upon the individual's emotional development. But who are more compassionate, men or women ? The answer to this question has been sought by an investigation carried out by the Department of Communication of the California State University (USA) (Salazar, 2016).

The study involved 613 university students, aged between 18 and 42 years, of which 310 were women. They were all given a set of standardised questionnaires. To measure levels of compassion the Compassion Scale was used (Pommier, Neff & Toth-Kiraly, 2020); to assess the level of tension when communicating the Personal Report of Communication Apprehension (Levine & McCroskey, 1990) was used; to assess the level of neuroticism the Hypersensitive Narcissism Scale (Hendin & Cheek, 1997) was used and finally, to assess the level of verbal aggressiveness the Verbal Aggressiveness Scale (Infante & Wigley, 1986) was used.

The results showed significant gender differences in terms of compassion, it being higher in the women participants. Significant differences were also found in the level of tension in communication and verbal aggressiveness, which were both higher in men. No gender differences were shown in terms of levels of narcissism. In terms of interaction, it was found that the more compassionate the participant, the lower the levels of communication tension, verbal aggressiveness and narcissism

Returning to the subject of the attacks on Asian people, in some cases these were related to the fact that they were wearing masks for no apparent reason, due to the fact that they were following the recommendations of their own governments, even though they were not in their own country.

In some European countries, due to the scarcity of masks, it has been recommended that masks are only worn if the individual has symptoms in order to not spread the disease, therefore on seeing an Asian person on the street in a mask, it could be easy to assume they are infected, thus filling people with fear and leading them to attack or drive the person away (@Cahora, 2020) (See Illustration 27).

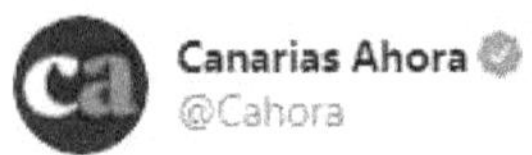

🚔🚔 Arranca de un mordisco un trozo de oreja a un hombre que le recriminó un comentario xenófobo hacia un trabajador chino #SUCESOS #GRANCANARIA eldiario.es/canariasahora/...

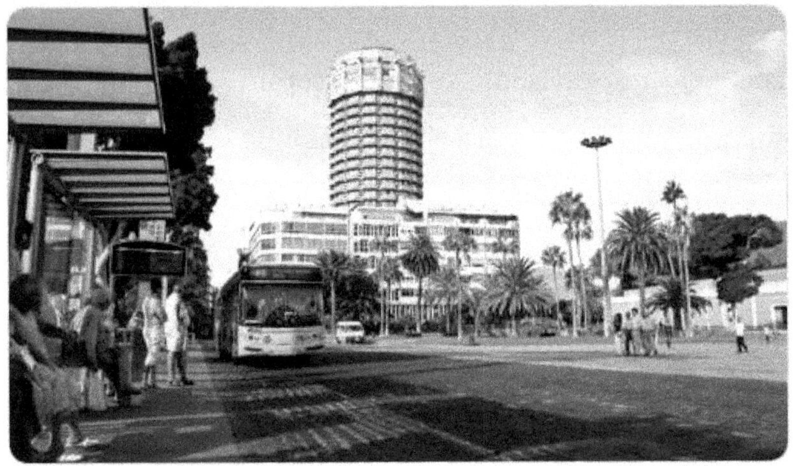

11:26 a. m. · 3 mar. 2020 · Twitter Web App

Illustration 27. Tweet – Xenophobia towards China

[A piece of a man's ear is bitten off for the condemnation of a xenophobic comment made against a Chinese worker]

Such behaviour is a form of aggression motivated by feelings of a fear of infection and 'defence' of one's own territory, belligerent behaviour which in any other circumstance would be unacceptable but, when fear is implanted in a society, anything becomes 'justified'.

There is a discussion in the field of behavioural science

about the essence of the nature of a human being; is it a rational animal who sometimes has flashes of emotion, or an emotional animal who voluntarily renounces that part to be governed by social norms and logic? That is to say, is a human being eminently emotional or eminently reflective?

There have been three traditionally adopted positions as to whether emotions predominate over reason in the guidance of human behaviour. There are those who argue that, in certain circumstances, emotions block and cancel cognition, precisely those abilities and capacities which characterise a human being, as compared to the simple mathematical or categorical processing of data by a computer. This would be an evolutionary mechanism, in which emotions are prioritised over cognition, useful when responding to danger, where the person runs away or remains paralysed – in both instances before they are able to 'think'. This may be observed, for instance, in the phenomenon of the stampede, which is the cause of so many problems at large events, where, if appropriate measures are not taken, any problem, such as an explosion of a firecracker, can generate a flood of people, all trying to escape from the place at the same time.

A mass movement led by the 'every man for himself' principle, leading to people being inadvertently trampled on, due to the fact that the crowd is not thinking, but simply acting to get away from the danger as quickly as possible. If any of those who managed to flee were asked why they ran, they would not be able to give a coherent answer, just that they did so because they felt their life could be in danger (@PanamericanaTV, 2020) (See Illustration 28).

panamericanatv
@PanamericanaTV
Níger: estampida humana durante entrega de alimentos deja al menos 20 muertos ptv.pe/286909

INTERNACIONALES
http://ptv.pe/286909
6:10 p. m. · 18 feb. 2020 · PanamericanaTV

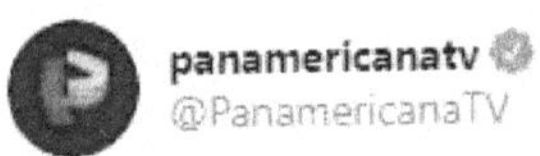

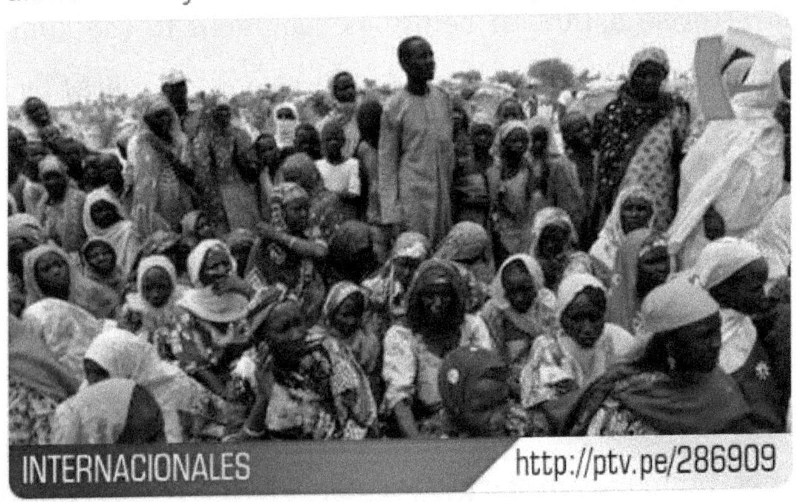

Illustration 28. Tweet – Human Stampede

[Niger: human stampede during the arrival of a food delivery leaves at least 20 dead]

This is something that, far from being anecdotal, costs the lives of hundreds of pilgrims each year when they gather in Mecca to pray, despite continuous security changes in attempts to prevent it.

The opposite standpoint argues that what defines the human, making him different from animals, are the higher cognitive processes, relegating the emotions to secondary, irrational and almost always incorrect processes, typical of animals. Such viewpoint suggests that human decision-making is carried out in a cost-benefit calculated way, in the manner of a supercomputer. This way of thinking is based on the premise that ability to put reason before impulsive behaviour in decision-making is a developing skill, and, by the same token, people

who do not stop to think may be trained to put in writing the pros and cons of each decision, and then adopt the one which offers the most benefits.

In fact, computers were initially developed to facilitate such calculations, due to the multitude of variables that had to be taken into account. Nowadays, artificial intelligence is sought to be creative rather than logical in order to approximate human intelligence.

The third approach is one which considers both processes as independent which, in certain circumstances, work together. Thanks to recent advances in the field of neuroscience, this standpoint is well supported. Based on this approach it may be concluded that human behaviour is sometimes guided by reasoning and at others by emotions.

In any event, what is clear is that the emotional world exists, is part of our self, and is reflected in all the decisions made on a daily basis, be they of minor or major importance.

Returning to the subject of fear, which is viewed as the generation of specific responses in an individual as a way of survival, one would not expect it to have any particular wider social consequences. However, data produced from the distant field of politics suggests otherwise, by way of studies in the field of political psychology concerning the understanding of how and why people vote the way they do.

Every election has its own peculiarities, sometimes with new agendas, candidates or parties, and in most cases they are usually limited to a few elections, although there are more in those systems where there is a 'second round', whereby candidates may only be chosen from parties that have obtained a minimum number of votes in the first round.

Psychologists who advise on electoral campaigns in order to optimise results analyse the different elections, as well as the way in which the population is 'responding', looking for relevant variables and patterns to help a candidate win in the next elections. Sometimes these are carried out in 'special' circumstances, which are usually one of a kind, so there is no prior knowledge available, as in the case of Spain's decision of whether or not to join NATO, and the United Kingdom's decision to leave the European Union, in what has become known as BREXIT. But did emotional aspects affect BREXIT? This question has been addressed by research undertaken by the Department of Psychology, Anglia Ruskin University; the Department of Clinical, Educational and Health Psychology, University of London (UK); together with the Centre for Psychology Medicine, Perdana University (Malaysia); and the Department of Leadership and Organizational Behaviour, Norwegian Business School (Norway) (Swami, V., Barron, D., Weis, L & Furnham, A., 2018).

The study involved 303 adults between the ages of 18 and 74 years of ages, of whom 92.4% were of 'white' descendancy, and 58.7% were female. All participants were interviewed three months before the voting took place and asked about their intention to vote; their identification with nationalist groups using the Collective Self-Esteem Scale (Luhtanen & Crocker, 1992); ; their perception regarding Muslim immigration; their belief in conspiracy theories about Islamophobia; on Islamophobia directly via the Islamophobia Scale (Lee, Gibbons, Thompson & Timani, 2009); ; their beliefs on conspiracy theories using the Generic Conspiracist Beliefs Scale (Brotherton, French & Pickering) ; and their tolerance to ambiguity using the Tolerance for Ambiguity Scale (Herman, Stevens, Bird, Mendenhall & Oddou, 2010).

The results showed a significant relationship between the belief in conspiracy theories and Islamophobia, that relationship being the mediating influence on how they would vote on leaving the European Union. Thus, the authors highlighted that in this study the participants' intention to vote was not guided by feelings of Euroscepticism or nationalism, but it was mediated by the fear generated by comparative theories regarding Islam. Therefore, according to the data presented, despite the fact that the voters should have been choosing whether or not they wanted to stay in the European Union, they were actually voting as to whether they wished to continue to take in Islamists, at a risk to their security and way of life, or not.

It is this fear, generated by the belief in conspiracy theories, which mobilised the electorate to say 'no' to Europe. There was no kind of rejection of Europe, its institutions or its population, neither was there any increased sentiments of patriotism or nationalism when the electorate was 'sold' campaigns in favour of the exit from the European Union (@RevistaSemana, 2020) (See Illustration 29). As this research shows, the fear of insecurity mobilised the electorate to choose the option which offered a priori more 'security' – a departure from Europe, in order to stop the massive influx of people with Islamic beliefs.

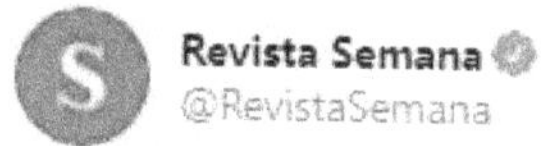

Un tribunal de Londres decidió este miércoles convocar al excanciller @BorisJohnson, candidato favorito para reemplazar a la primera ministra Theresa May, acusado de haber mentido deliberadamente durante la campaña del referéndum de 2016 sobre el Brexit bit.ly/2YQkOg4

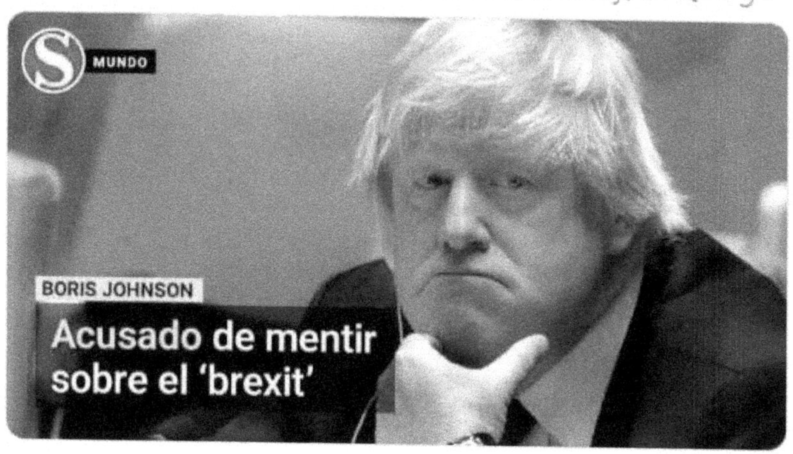

2:00 p. m. · 29 may. 2019 · TweetDeck

Illustration 29. Tweet – Manipulation of Brexit

[A London tribunal decided this Wednesday to summon the former chancellor, Boris Johnson, the favourite candidate to replace current prime minister Theresa May, who is accused of deliberately lying about Brexit during the referendum campaign of 2016]

In other words, and in accordance with that already discussed, it may be seen that fear is a primary emotion which can be generated and transmitted quickly, causing 'irrational' behaviour which may even go against established norms thus potentially endangering the integrity of society, e.g. in the demonstration of aggression towards Asian people by attributing responsibility to them for the spread of the virus throughout the world.

Whilst this explanation does not vindicate such behaviour, it does put into perspective why people with socially infected emotions may become aggressive in expressing their fears. Although this concerns a negative perspective, such contagion may also occur with regards positive emotions, as in the case of solidarity movements to which people 'sign up' without realising their motivations. They may simply think it is the right thing to do at the time, not realising their actions are due to emotional contagion.

It should be mentioned, regarding the subject of race

mentioned earlier, that biology now rules out the concept of different races, since there are insufficient genetic or phenotypic differences to support such a theory, which is now considered an ambiguous and misleading concept (@CRCiencia, 2018) (See Illustration 30).

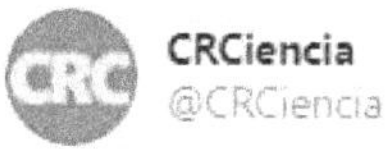

CRCiencia
@CRCiencia

La raza es una idea de agrupamiento social > desde la biología y la genética solo existe una única raza, la humana ow.ly/p5hV30mjU0k #Biologia

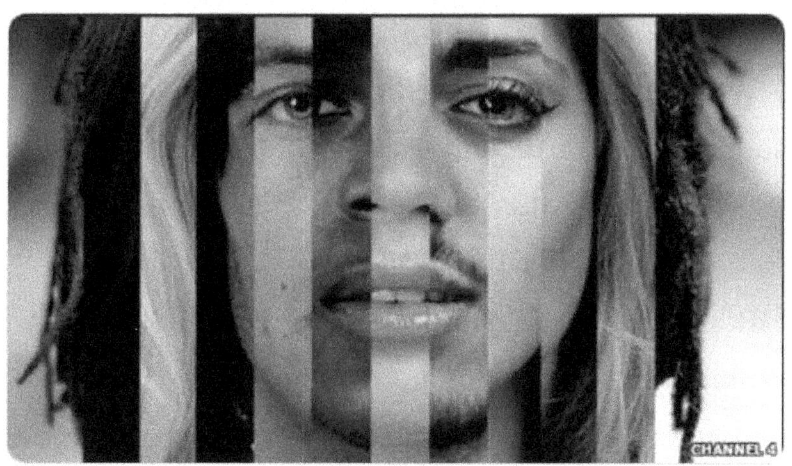

8:20 p. m. · 22 oct. 2018 · Hootsuite Inc.

Illustration 30. Tweet – Biology and Race

[Race is a social grouping concept > according to biology and genetics there is only one race, the human]

Although societies are usually made up of individuals with more or less similar genetic and physical characteristics, the factors which make them identify as a country or nation are the ideological aspects, such as beliefs, values and, of course, a shared culture.

Whilst it is true that shared 'traits' exist, due to belonging to the same species, most of these are mediated by culture which is learned from a young age, an aspect which becomes evident when travelling, in observing how, what is 'normal' or 'expected' in one location is not the same in another.

With regards emotions, there is some controversy as to whether they are universal or whether they vary dependent on locality, that is to say whether they are genetically or culturally based.

Regarding behaviour, it is widely accepted that learning plays a predominant role.

For example, it has been observed how the simplest of things, such as nodding the head to say yes, or moving it from side to side to say no, is not universal, since there exist many different variations dependent upon country, for instance in the case of Bulgaria (@RafaelPoulain, 2018) (See Illustration 31).

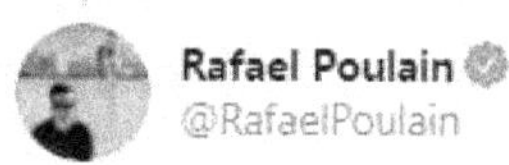

Rafael Poulain
@RafaelPoulain

En Bulgaria la gente mueve lo cabeza de arriba a abajo para decir "No" y de un lado a otro para decir "Sí".

#RaFacts

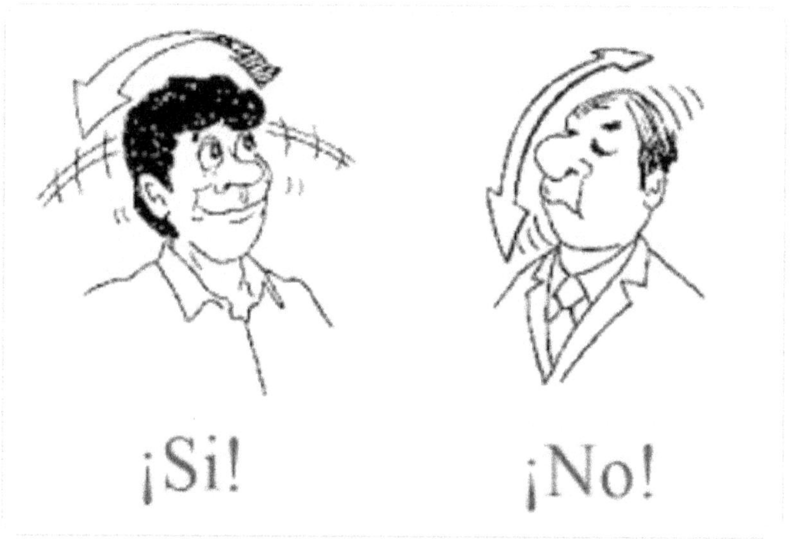

11:25 p. m. · 2 jul. 2018 · Twitter for iPhone

Illustration 31. Tweet - Idioms in Bulgaria

[In Bulgaria people nod their head to say "no" and from side to side to say "Yes".]

Framed within these cultural studies is the analysis of social components, such as the recognition of gestures or faces, which are essential in non-verbal communication. Although we have no difficulty in recognising the traits of a person from our own country, this becomes more difficult the further afield we travel, hence the expression 'all Chinese look the same', since we have particular difficulty in identifying both their expressive features and their face itself. But why do all Chinese people look the same to us? This question has been addressed by research undertaken by the Faculty of Psychology and Cognitive Science, East China Normal University; the Faculty of Education, Zhejiang University (China); together with the Department of Psychology, Humboldt State University (USA); and the Institute of Neuroscience and Psychology, University of Glasgow (UK) (Wang et al., 2019).

The investigation was carried out in three stages. In the first stage 50 men and 50 women were selected, all Chinese, and six photographs of their faces were taken, then 10 men and 22 women, all Chinese, evaluated the emotion of the faces, leaving only those who were neutral. Finally, 10 men and 10 women, all Chinese, identified up to 14 face traits on a Likert-type scale from 1 to 7, with 1 being low trait presence and 7 being high trait presence.

Results showed that there are two traits which explained 85% of the variance, the first being accessibility/valence, whilst the second was cordiality. Previous research has shown that the accessibility/valence trait tends to be used by the Western population, demonstrated in a friendly and 'harmless' face. Regarding the second trait, cordiality, this is not an element used in the distinguishing of faces by Westerners, but is a distinctive feature used in the processing of faces amongst Asians. In the light of the foregoing, it may be concluded that there is a cultural component in face processing which means that, in the differentiation of features, some will focus more on certain aspects than others.

Having commented on the 'difficulty' of distinguishing between people of another race, and even between populations with similar traits, such as Filipino, Chinese or Korean people who share similar complexions and eye shape, it is worth analysing the problem of violence against these groups.

In this regard an analysis would need to be carried out, taking into account the personality or mental health of the assailant, in addition to their sociodemographic characteristics, work and even social relations. Similarly, their closest environment would need to be analysed in order to 'understand' what the trigger is for the attacks on said population.

Much has been said about hatred between races, involving factors associated with immigration or an erroneous feeling of national 'protection', but these have all been conjecture. There have also been accusations of a political nature, in the sense of pointing out one or another as being 'responsible' for certain extremist feelings.

Some analysts have indicated how opinions have been radicalised on social networks, and concretised in the identification of particular ways of how to attack, leaving the more theoretical discussions to one side. Such concretisation could therefore have been the 'source of inspiration' for some of these aggressors. Therefore, without reaching any conclusions, the prevailing ideas for the explanation of such behaviour are both political and technological in nature. But do social networks serve radicalism? This question has been addressed in a study by Princeton University and Ithaca College; with the School of Computing, George Mason University and the Indiana University (USA); together with Qatar University (Qatar) (Alizadeh, Weber, Cioffi-Revilla, Fortunato & Macy 2019).

This particular research is based on postings on Twitter, one of the most active social networks in terms of expression of emotions. Included in the study were 10,000 user accounts, half of whom self-identified themselves as liberal and half as conservatives. An analysis was made of their tweets, excluding links and Retweets, and classifying them according to the level of 'extremism' contained within, comparing the ones written by those with the most and least extreme same political opinion, versus those of the other political opinion.

The results indicated that those who are more extremist, regardless of their political persuasion, share less positive and more negative emotions concerning non-extremists, although the difference was not significant. The results also showed that liberals tend to express themselves more anxiously than conservatives. Amongst the limitations of the study was the fact that the authors excluded Retweets, i.e. those not originally written by the participants.

This meant exclusion of much of the political communication, broadly based on the 'repetition' of the slogans of opinion leaders, whether they be the politicians themselves, or the campaign personnel. Furthermore, when selecting the participants, it was assumed that each account belonged to a single person. However, this would not always be the case since, on occasions, individuals, particularly the most active ones, have several accounts via which they circulate their ideas and emotions, therefore by not controlling this aspect, the results obtained may have been magnified. However, despite the foregoing, such a study remains an innovative way in which to tackle the problem of the disclosure of extremism on social networks.

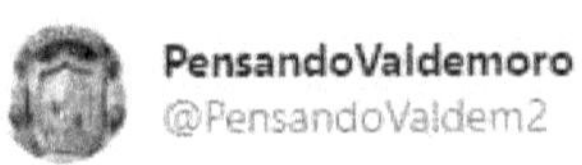

Cierran los comercios "chinos" de #Valdemoro. La llegada del #coronavirus a nuestra ciudad parece estar detrás de la causa de este cierre. Los pocos que permanecen abiertos atiende a sus clientes con mascarilas

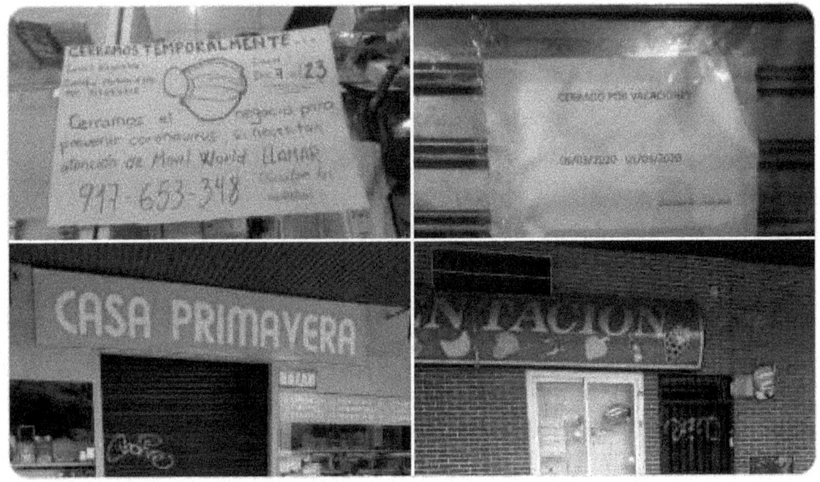

Telenoticias Telemadrid y 9 más

9:43 a. m. · 7 mar. 2020 · Twitter Web App

<u>Illustration 32. Tweet - Closure of Chinese Shops</u>

[Closure of the Chinese shops of #Valdemoro. The arrival of coronavirus to our city seems to be behind the reason for this closure. The few that remain open serve their clients in masks]

During the times of COVID-19, Chinese communities in different countries have asked to not be stigmatised, insulted or attacked. They have been suffering this kind of harassment due to accusations of being responsible for a disease which started thousands of miles from where they live. In some countries they have suffered acts of vandalism to their business establishments, leading them to close temporarily in order to prevent escalation of the violence against them (PensandoValdem, 2020) (See Illustration 32), and also to 'isolate' themselves away from the population. In a similar way, in some schools, Chinese parents decided not to take their children to school in order to avoid any 'misunderstandings'.

List of Illustrations

@Cahora. (2020). Canarias Ahora en Twitter: "?? Arranca de un mordisco un trozo de oreja a un hombre que le recriminó un comentario xenófobo hacia un trabajador chino #SUCESOS #GRANCANARIA https://t.co/Q38MF6fP8T https://t.co/rwZc8HdH7H" / Twitter. Retrieved April 4, 2020, from https://twitter.com/Cahora/status/1234787142020325376

@CRCiencia. (2018). CRCiencia en Twitter: "La raza es una idea de agrupamiento social > desde la biología y la genética solo existe una única raza, la humana https://t.co/iqskDVs7ad #Biologia https://t.co/3hWJmhMWx4" / Twitter. Retrieved April 4, 2020, from https://twitter.com/CRCiencia/status/1054437251889934337

@informativost5. (2020). Informativos Telecinco en Twitter: "Temor al coronavirus: le propinan un puñetazo por defender a su amiga china https://t.co/ogWSEkZS71" / Twitter. Retrieved April 4, 2020, from https://twitter.com/informativost5/status/1231573028691152896

@maestrocarlosef. (2019). PRoFe CaRLoS en Twitter: "Y llegó el día, hoy 12 de noviembre de 2019 celebramos el Día contra la obesidad infantil desde el proyecto del @CaMiNoPieFCiToS con la campaña DA UN SALTO CONTRA LA OBESIDAD INFANTIL en la que llenaremos los centros educativos d. Retrieved April 4, 2020, from https://twitter.com/maestrocarlosef/status/1194108678288396291

@minsalud. (2020). Ministerio de Salud en Twitter: "El país se mantiene a cero casos sospechosos y cero casos confirmados de coronavirus (COVID-19). Unámonos a la prevención de esta enfermedad siguiendo estas recomendaciones: ? https://t.co/7S4oeZJ9cb" / Twitter. Retrieved April 4, 2020, from https://twitter.com/minsalud/status/123395838071004 3651

@Newtral. (2020). Newtral en Twitter: "Mascarillas, viseras e incluso respiradores. Miles de personas con impresoras 3D están intentando ayudar al personal sanitario creando material EPI en sus casas. https://t.co/lSVH3rjmMF https://t.co/peyLSQDWDP" / Twitter. Retrieved April 4, 2020, from https://twitter.com/Newtral/status/1244782470580576 257

@PanamericanaTV. (2020). Panamericanatv en Twitter: "Níger: estampida humana durante entrega de alimentos deja al menos 20 muertos https://t.co/I1sVi3aBjb https://t.co/tZAld1tAMb" / Twitter. Retrieved April 4, 2020, from https://twitter.com/PanamericanaTV/status/12298154 75586113536

@PensandoValdem2. (2020). PensandoValdemoro en Twitter: "Cierran los comercios "chinos" de #Valdemoro. La llegada del #coronavirus a nuestra ciudad parece estar detrás de la causa de este cierre. Los pocos que permanecen abiertos atiende a sus clientes con mascarilas https://t.co/. Retrieved April 4, 2020, from https://twitter.com/PensandoValdem2/status/1236210 961939337217

@RafaelPoulain. (2018). Rafael Poulain en Twitter: "En Bulgaria la gente mueve lo cabeza de arriba a abajo para decir 'No' y de un lado a otro para decir 'Sí'. #RaFacts https://t.co/EFwRsDnknm" / Twitter. Retrieved April 4, 2020, from https://twitter.com/RafaelPoulain/status/10138963434 40449537

@Renzo_Utili. (2020). Renzo en Twitter: “??? ITALIA aisla en rígida Cuarentena a 16 Millones de personas, nadie podrá salir o entrar solo por motivos muy urgentes: mapa https://t.co/jOCVj3DtrS” / Twitter. Retrieved April 4, 2020, from https://twitter.com/Renzo_Utili/status/1236620725018116101

@RevistaSemana. (2020). Revista Semana en Twitter: "Un tribunal de Londres decidió este miércoles convocar al excanciller @BorisJohnson, candidato favorito para reemplazar a la primera ministra Theresa May, acusado de haber mentido deliberadamente durante la campaña del referénd. Retrieved April 4, 2020, from https://twitter.com/RevistaSemana/status/1133704540409040896

@RSF_ES. (2020). RSF España en Twitter: "COSTA DE MARFIL | Fuertes multas para dos periodistas por publicar “noticias falsas”. RSF expresa su preocupación por este paso atrás en un país que llevaba varios años mejorando en libertad de prensa // Inglés, web de @RSF_inter h. Retrieved April 4, 2020, from https://twitter.com/RSF_ES/status/1246139604132077570

@sanidadgob. (2020a). Ministerio de Sanidad en Twitter: "?La limpieza adecuada y frecuente de las manos es más eficaz que el uso de guantes, porque: ➡Usarlos durante mucho tiempo hace que se ensucien y puedan contaminarse ➡Quitarse los guantes sin contaminarse las manos no. Retrieved April 4, 2020, from https://twitter.com/sanidadgob/status/1245983562509307904

@sanidadgob. (2020b). Ministerio de Sanidad en Twitter: "Nuestras vidas han cambiado de la noche a la mañana con la crisis del #COVID19 en el mundo Es importante: ✅Reconoce tus emociones ✅Genera una rutina

✅Céntrate en lo que puedes hacer ✅Cuídate ✅Desconecta ✅Mantén con. Retrieved April 4, 2020, from https://twitter.com/sanidadgob/status/1243568462808731658

@SeremiSaludRM. (2020). Seremi de Salud RM en Twitter: "#CuidémonosEntreTodos . Respeta la cuarentena en tu hogar. Hazlo por ti y tu familia. Denuncia en ?? https://t.co/TMt3CLXiGV para quienes no lo respeten. https://t.co/juLHxEDxEz" / Twitter. Retrieved April 4, 2020, from https://twitter.com/SeremiSaludRM/status/1243929339248300032

@shildalys. (2020). ☪hildaly☪ en Twitter: "#coronoavirus 24 d enero 2020: #China pone en cuarentena 8 ciudades más en la provincia d Hubei, atrapando a 35 millones de residentes en sus ciudades. Al cierre d esta edición, 2019-nCoV ha matado a 26 pacientes, todos en China. En. Retrieved April 4, 2020, from https://twitter.com/shildalys/status/1220867654560468998

@SilenciosoVox. (2020). Vamos a vencer al virus● ?? en Twitter: "Holanda eres de PM https://t.co/N13ErnNhJO" / Twitter. Retrieved April 4, 2020, from https://twitter.com/SilenciosoVox/status/1243623205908201472

@VicentGrimalt. (2020). Vicent Grimalt en Twitter: "Finalmente, la crisis por el coronavirus nos obliga, por razones obvias de prevención, a aplazar la celebración de las Fallas también en #Dénia, según ha acordado el Govern de la Generalitat. Entendemos la decepción y la preocu. Retrieved April 4, 2020, from https://twitter.com/VicentGrimalt/status/123749963678089216

References

Alizadeh, M., Weber, I., Cioffi-Revilla, C., & Fortunato & Macy, S. F. (2019). Psychology and morality of political extremists: evidence from Twitter language analysis of alt-right and Antifa. *Springer*. Retrieved from https://link.springer.com/article/10.1140/epjds/s13688-019-0193-9

Beißert, H. M., & Hasselhorn, M. (2016). Individual Differences in Moral Development: Does Intelligence Really Affect Children's Moral Reasoning and Moral Emotions? *Frontiers in Psychology*, *7*(DEC), 1961. https://doi.org/10.3389/fpsyg.2016.01961

Brotherton, R., French, C. C., & Pickering, A. D. (2013). Measuring Belief in Conspiracy Theories: The Generic Conspiracist Beliefs Scale. *Frontiers in Psychology*, *4*(MAY), 279. https://doi.org/10.3389/fpsyg.2013.00279

Dungan, J. A., Young, L., & Waytz, A. (2019). The power of moral concerns in predicting whistleblowing decisions. *Journal of Experimental Social Psychology*, *85*, 103848. https://doi.org/10.1016/j.jesp.2019.103848

Egloff, B., Schwerdtfeger, A., & Schmukle, S. C. (2005). Temporal stability of the Implicit Association Test-Anxiety. *Journal of Personality Assessment*, *84*(1), 82–88. https://doi.org/10.1207/s15327752jpa8401_14

Greenwald, A. G., McGhee, D. E., & Schwartz, J. L. K. (1998). Measuring individual differences in implicit cognition: The implicit association test. *Journal of Personality and Social Psychology*, *74*(6), 1464–1480. https://doi.org/10.1037/0022-3514.74.6.1464

Hendin, H. M., & Cheek, J. M. (1997). Assessing hypersensitive narcissism: A reexamination of Murray's Narcism Scale. *Journal of Research in Personality*, *31*(4), 588–599.

Herman, J. L., Stevens, M. J., Bird, A., Mendenhall, M., & Oddou, G. (2010). The Tolerance for Ambiguity Scale: Towards a more refined measure for international management research. *International Journal of*

Intercultural Relations, *34*(1), 58–65. https://doi.org/10.1016/j.ijintrel.2009.09.004

Holland, P. C., & Gallagher, M. (1993). Effects of Amygdala Central Nucleus Lesions on Blocking and Unblocking. *Behavioral Neuroscience*, *107*(2), 235–245. https://doi.org/10.1037/0735-7044.107.2.235

Holland, P. C., & Gallagher, M. (1999, February 1). Amygdala circuitry in attentional and representational processes. *Trends in Cognitive Sciences*, Vol. 3, pp. 65–73. https://doi.org/10.1016/S1364-6613(98)01271-6

Hübner, G., Mohs, A., & Petersen, L. E. (2014). The Role of Attitude Strength in Predicting Organ Donation Behaviour by Implicit and Explicit Attitude Measures. *Open Journal of Medical Psychology*, *03*(05), 355–363. https://doi.org/10.4236/ojmp.2014.35037

Infante, D. A., & Wigley, C. J. (1986). Verbal aggressiveness: An interpersonal model and measure. *Communication Monographs*, *53*(1), 61–69. https://doi.org/10.1080/03637758609376126

Kohlberg, L. (1969). *Stage and sequence; The cognitive-developmental approach to socialization.*

Lang, P., Bradley, M., Cuthbert, B., Lang, P., Bradley, M., Cuthbert, B., ... Simons, R. (1997, January 1). *Motivated attention: affect, activation and action.*

Lazar, J. N., & Pearlman-Avnion, S. (2014). Effect of Affect Induction Method on Emotional Valence and Arousal. *Psychology*, *05*(07), 595–601. https://doi.org/10.4236/psych.2014.57070

Lee, S. A., Gibbons, J. A., Thompson, J. M., & Timani, H. S. (2009). The Islamophobia scale: Instrument development and initial validation. *Ethics and Behavior*, *19*(2), 92–105. https://doi.org/10.1080/10508610802711137

Levine, T. R., & Mccroskey, J. C. (1990). Measuring Trait Communication Apprehension: A Test Of Rival Measurement Models Of The Prca-24. *Communication Monographs*, *57*(1), 62–72. https://doi.org/10.1080/03637759009376185

Li, M., Taylor, E. G., Atkins, K. E., Chapman, G. B., & Galvani, A. P. (2016). Stimulating influenza vaccination via prosocial motives. *PLoS ONE, 11*(7), e0159780. https://doi.org/10.1371/journal.pone.0159780

Luhtanen, R., & Crocker, J. (1992). A collective self-esteem scale: Self-evaluation of one's social identity. *Personality and Social Psychology Bulletin, 18*(3), 302–318. https://doi.org/10.1177/0146167292183006

Norton, M. I., Mochon, D., & Ariely, D. (2012). The IKEA effect: When labor leads to love. *Journal of Consumer Psychology, 22*(3), 453–460. https://doi.org/10.1016/j.jcps.2011.08.002

Phelps, E. A., O'Connor, K. J., Cunningham, W. A., Funayama, E. S., Gatenby, J. C., Gore, J. C., & Banaji, M. R. (2000). Performance on indirect measures of race evaluation predicts amygdala activation. *Journal of Cognitive Neuroscience, 12*(5), 729–738. https://doi.org/10.1162/089892900562552

Pommier, E., Neff, K. D., & Tóth-Király, I. (2020). The Development and Validation of the Compassion Scale. *Assessment, 27*(1), 21–39.

Salazar, L. R. (2016). The relationship between compassion, interpersonal communication apprehension, narcissism and verbal aggressiveness. *The Journal of Happiness and Well-Being, 4*(1), 1–14. Retrieved from http://www.journalofhappiness.net/article/the-relationship-between-compassion-interpersonal-communication-apprehension-narcissism-and-verbal-aggressiveness

Swami, V., Barron, D., Weis, L.& Furnham, A. (2018). To Brexit or not to Brexit: The roles of Islamophobia, conspiracist beliefs, and integrated threat in voting intentions for the United Kingdom European Union. *British Journal of Psychology, 109*(1), 156–179. https://doi.org/10.1111/bjop.12252

van den Bos, R., Jolles, J. W., & Homberg, J. (2013, June 5). Social modulation of decision-making: A cross-species review. *Frontiers in Human Neuroscience*, Vol. 7, p. 301.

https://doi.org/10.3389/fnhum.2013.00301

Wang, H., Han, C., Hahn, A. C., Fasolt, V., Morrison, D. K., Holzleitner, I. J., ... Jones, B. C. (2019). A data-driven study of Chinese participants' social judgments of Chinese faces. *PLoS ONE*, *14*(1). https://doi.org/10.1371/journal.pone.0210315

Weiß, R. H., Osterland, J., & Cattell, R. B. (1977). *Grundintelligenztest Skala 1: CFT 1*. Westermann.

Wukmir, V. J. (1967). *Emoción y sufrimiento: endoantropología elemental*. Editorial Labor.

Chapter 3. Mental Health and Lockdown

The implementation of lockdown has proved to be one of the most high-profile and unpopular measures ever, and never more so when, for the first time in history, the Chinese government closed down one of its provinces, preventing the free movement of its inhabitants, and dictating that they remain locked in their homes, only to be allowed out to get food for themselves.

These were unprecedented measures to date, but they were justified by the health authorities as a way to combat the spread of COVID-19, thereby reducing the possibility of infecting other people. Furthermore, in this way the rest of the country was 'protected' from the spread of the disease. A method which was also adopted by Italy when the number of infected rose uncontrollably, and later in many other countries, to a lesser or greater degree.

Putting ourselves, for a moment, in the position of somebody in that particular locality, we realise that, overnight, measures have been put in place limiting our movements and confining us to our own home for days and days, without knowing for how long the situation will last, and even if the measures will prove effective. Furthermore, only those with financial resources or who work online will avoid the dilemma which others face, when their money runs out and they are unable to work because everything is closed. But this is the situation which millions of inhabitants have confronted for months, with the added uncertainty of not knowing how the virus is transmitted or whether they themselves are infected or not. An ongoing stressful situation which, dependent upon each individual's psychological makeup, will affect each one differently, and which, in some cases, will have medium to long term consequences which will continue after lockdown is over.

It is therefore predicted that a greater number of cases of depression or post -traumatic stress disorder will occur in this population, compared to those who did not have to undergo home confinement. Similar was observed in 2003, amongst those who isolated in cases of Severe Acute Respiratory Syndrome, which is from the same family as the coronavirus, and which causes severe pneumonia (Luna, 2020). Recommendations are therefore being made by international agencies and professional associations of psychologists, for the preservation of the mental health of those who have to be confined to their homes for months.

Attempts have been made to keep people occupied with leisure activities, along with the recommendation of age-appropriate advice for the leading of an orderly life in terms of food, personal care and sport. Everyone has surely heard of the well-known phrase 'healthy mind in a healthy body', which means that in order to have adequate mental health the physical body must also be taken care of, an aspect which is often not taken into account. But when the time comes when we do want to exercise, a number of questions arise. Should we exercise daily? What type of exercise would be the most convenient? How much time should be devoted to exercise? These are typical questions which need addressing.

Although prior to the appearance of COVID-19, when someone was asked on the street by interviewers collecting information on health habits, lack of time was the main reason attributed to the fact of not carrying out any daily physical exercise, in the current circumstances of lockdown, time is no longer an excuse, as reflected in the official recommendations (@ConsejoCOLEF, 2020) (See Illustration 33).

If one thing is clear, it is the many benefits of daily exercise at a moderate level, either in oxygenating the body, or helping tone and maintain adequate flexibility. But does exercise really help the brain? This question has been addressed by research undertaken in a study by Shanghai Punan Hospital; the Shanghai University of Sport and the Tianjin University of Sport (China) (Pi et al., 2019).

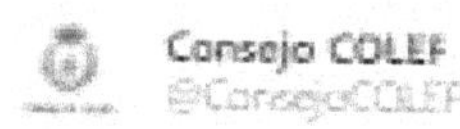

.@deportegob y @ConsejoCOLEF recomiendan seguir manteniendo estilos de vida activos durante el confinamiento.

Si tienes dudas sobre cómo entrenar en casa, contacta con profesionales cualificados/as del deporte.

#YoMeMuevoEnCasa #YoEntrenoEnCasa

consejo-colef.es/recomendacione...

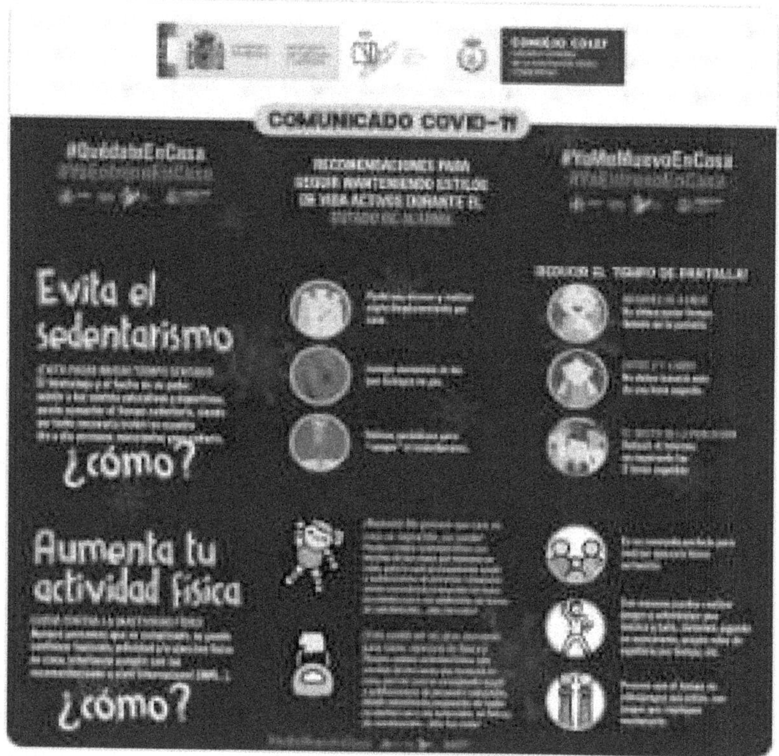

5:10 p. m. · 31 mar. 2020 · Twitter for Advertisers.

Illustration 33. Tweet – Sport in Lockdown

[@deporte.gob y @ConsejoCOLEF recommends continuing the maintenance of healthy lifestyles during lockdown. If you have doubts about training at home, contact qualified sport professionals.]

The study involved 46 boys, aged between 19 and 22 years, 21 of whom were basketball professionals who trained for six hours a day on average five days a week, and the rest (the control group) were university students who did not habitually practice any sport. They all underwent a diffusion tensor analysis to examine density of the white matter, which allows interconnectivity between areas, regions and hemispheres of the brain.

The results of the comparison between athletes and non-athletes demonstrated that the experts had shorter routes between regions, making it easier for them to be more efficient in their performance. It was also observed that the circuits involved in tasks associated with sports practice were especially optimised for attention and visual processing, fundamental aspects in this particular sport which, not only consists of shooting a ball into a basket, for which good vision is essential, but within the game, the ball is continually passed to teammates or removed from opponents, therefore attention must be paid to one's teammates' signals, the coach's instructions, and the trajectory of the ball in opponents' hands in order to intercept them. Furthermore, the aforementioned results were significantly related to the number of years of training, hence the more years of training the higher the brain performance.

It may therefore be concluded that one does not need to be a professional athlete for daily practice, even moderate, to help the brain in the optimisation of its various processes. It is therefore advisable to carry out some form of activity with which to improve and tone the body, in addition to maintaining a 'healthy' and optimised brain, thus reducing the hours spent in sedentary activity, which is associated with specific health problems, and which exercise can prevent.

Emotions in Lockdown

If anything has characterised Western society, particularly in the last decade, it has been the pursuit of happiness. To this end, hundreds of self-help manuals have been written in the teaching of how to discover personal happiness.

Although every author defines it differently and establishes a different 'path' to achieve it, they all agree that the achievement of happiness is a social necessity, a social norm to which everyone should subscribe. But who wouldn't want to be happy?

There are many social demands surrounding the establishment of a 'good life' whereby an individual may consider it is not enough to just have a job, a house or a car. But when circumstances change, such as the current implementation of lockdown measures, prior wishes and desires may seem 'unrealistic', and the uncertainty surrounding the disease and what will happen next takes its toll, leading us to wonder, could the achievement of happiness we have been pursuing for so long lead to depression? An answer to this question has been sought by a study undertaken by the School of Psychology, University of New South Wales (Australia) and the Department of Psychology, KU Leuven University (Belgium) (Bastian et al, 2015).

The study involved 200 Belgian university students, ranging in age from 17 to 24 years of age, of whom 110 were women, drawn from a sample of 786 volunteers. For all of them social expectations were evaluated, particularly with regard to negative emotions such as loneliness, depression, sadness or anxiety. The presence of depressive symptoms was measured using the standardised Center for Epidemiological Studies Scale (Radloff, 1977), and the level of perceived loneliness was evaluated by the UCLA Loneliness Scale (Russell, 1996). In addition, all the participants underwent a situation where they were emotionally manipulated, making the student feel either better or worse about themself.

The results showed that those students with higher social expectations of achieving happiness were the ones who were the worst at accepting failure, causing them feelings of loneliness and depression. On the other hand, students with low social expectations of achieving happiness were the most tolerant of the fact of not achieving it, and they did not present such marked feelings of loneliness and depression.

These results suggest the need for reflection upon social demands and how at times one may, instead of facilitating the path to happiness, hinder it by asking for more than what is personally achievable, resulting in a 'social failure' and leading to negative feelings which may cause depression.

With the current situation of many countries being in lockdown, some people who have lost their jobs experience internalised demands creating negative feelings and thoughts of personal failure, because they are continuing to measure themselves on the same pre-lockdown 'social success' scale. This situation has affected workers with temporary contracts or who, due to the nature of their work, are unable to work remotely. The exacerbation of the difficult conditions in which they live, creates a trigger for mental health problems, which may start with symptoms of depression coupled with a strong feeling of personal unhappiness (@diarodeburgos, 2020) (See Illustration 34).

An important and fundamental variable in relating life experience to emotions is Emotional Intelligence which, if formed adequately during childhood, allows an individual to possess the necessary tools to face any frustration caused if the social expectation of happiness is not achieved.

As noted, happiness is intrinsically related to emotions. But what happens when an individual is subjected to emotional disturbance?

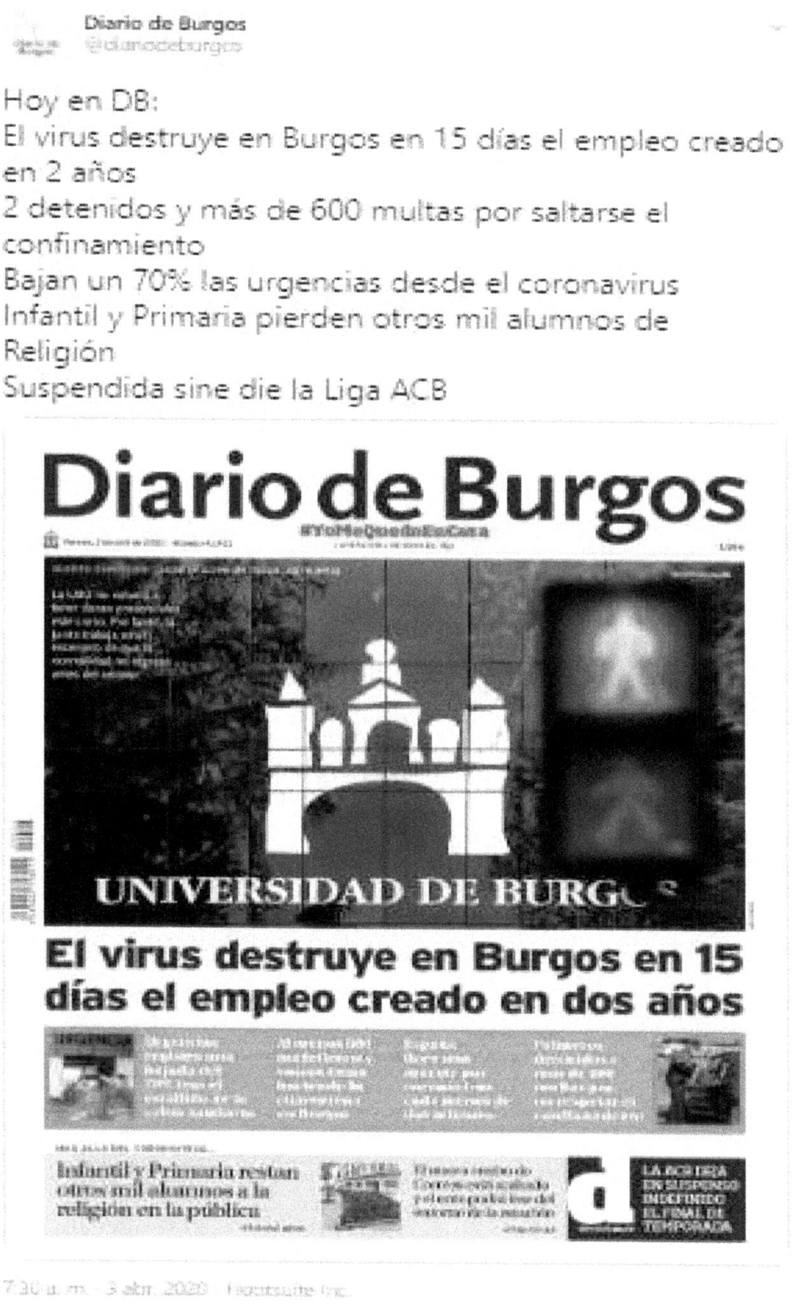

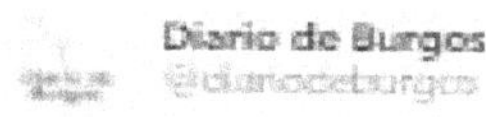

Hoy en DB:
El virus destruye en Burgos en 15 días el empleo creado en 2 años
2 detenidos y más de 600 multas por saltarse el confinamiento
Bajan un 70% las urgencias desde el coronavirus
Infantil y Primaria pierden otros mil alumnos de Religión
Suspendida sine die la Liga ACB

Diario de Burgos

#YoMeQuedoEnCasa

UNIVERSIDAD DE BURG

El virus destruye en Burgos en 15 días el empleo creado en dos años

Infantil y Primaria restan otros mil alumnos a la religión en la pública

LA ACB DEJA EN SUSPENSO INDEFINIDO EL FINAL DE TEMPORADA

7:30 a. m. · 3 abr. 2020 · Hootsuite Inc.

Illustration 34. Tweet – Unemployment in the face of Lockdown

Psychological Aspects in time of Pandemic

[Today in DB: In Burgos in 15 days the virus has destroyed jobs created over 2 years. 2 arrested and more than 600 fines issued for breaking of lockdown. 70% decrease in emergencies from coronavirus. Infant and Primary Schools lose another 1000 students of religion. La Liga ACB suspended sine die]

One's state of mind is the way in which one copes with daily activities and how one responds to any difficulties which may arise. The healthiest way is to adapt the state of mind to the specific circumstances, so at one moment a certain level of higher activity may be required, in giving a quick or energetic response, whilst at others they should be calm and slow. Therefore, everyone, throughout the day tends to go through almost every mood, with moments of lesser or greater intensity of personal activation, dependent upon the circumstances surrounding the individual.

However, when these states are altered, the individual responds in an imbalanced way to the requirements of the moment, i.e. in an inappropriate way, either with over-activity or inactivity, and contrary to what the current circumstances require. This will not only jeopardise the effectiveness of any work being carried out, but will also affect social, family and partner relationships.

These mood alterations may become ‘chronic’, causing the individual to maintain a continuous high level of activation, taking a toll on their health and causing irritability, rudeness and even aggressiveness, as may be observed in anxiety disorders where there is a continuous high level of activation not justified by the circumstances. When low activation responses become chronic, social, family and personal relationships will be impaired, but in this instance by excessive passivity which may result in inaction and absolute dependence upon others to carry out the simplest of tasks. This is what happens in major depressive disorder, where a relaxed and paused state becomes chronic, becoming part of the individual’s way of behaving.

These are the most frequent events involved in the emergence of mood disorders, although it is possible for a combination of both states to occur, classified as bipolar disorder, where moods switch from depressive to manic, and these changes of mood, which are out of step with the current circumstances, predominate. The sudden changes in state, without prior warning, and the intensity of some episodes, whether manic or depressive, may disconcert and even confuse those close to the sufferer. Although there are specific treatments in the control of these symptoms, allowing sufferers a longer period of stability, they are often abandoned by the patients. Believing that they are 'cured' or that they 'no longer need them' are the main motivations for stopping the medication. But how do patients with bipolar disorder experience their disorder? This question has been addressed in a study undertaken by the Department of Psychology, Kumaun University (India) (Chandola, 2016).

The study involved 40 patients diagnosed with bipolar disorder and 40 without (control group), and all of them were asked to complete the Dimension Personality Inventory (Bhargawa, 2012).

The results showed significant differences in gender (highest in women); in age (higher incidence amongst adults aged between 40 to 50 years versus young people aged between 20 to 30 years); but no significant differences in personality were found between the assessment of patients with bipolar disorder and the control group.

The authors of the study pointed out that these findings were unexpected because, unlike other disorders where symptoms may be less evident, but the patient is aware of and actually suffers from his illness, in the case of bipolar disorder there are very obvious dual symptoms evident, yet the situation does not appear to impact upon their personality.

Suffering from this disorder in a situation such as

lockdown, where the patient is confined for days and days can lead to a series of problems. The patient may abandon their treatment, leading to an increase in symptoms which will, in turn, affect other family members or carers who will also suffer if the patient experiences manic episodes due to lack of medicine (@ma_purity, 2020) (See Illustration 35).

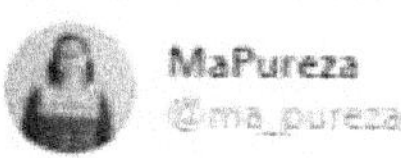

Hoy, en el Día Mundial del Trastorno Bipolar, hagamos conciencia sobre esta enfermedad. El aislamiento puede ser desafiante para muchos, pero es un reto para aquellos que tienen enfermedades mentales. Tengamos empatía con aquellos que las sufren.

(📷bit.ly/2Uxxiu1)

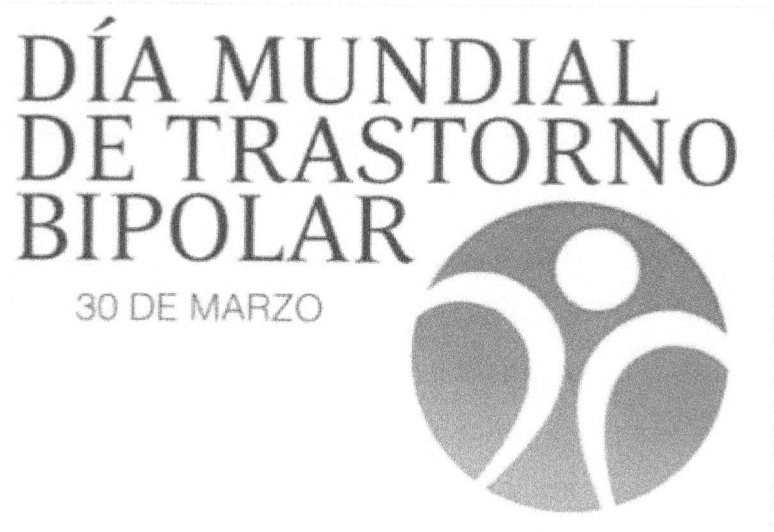

12:27 a. m. · 31 mar. 2020 · Twitter for iPhone

Illustration 35. Tweet- Bipolar in lockdown

[Today, on World Bipolar Day, we are raising awareness of this illness. Isolation can be difficult for many, but it is a real challenge for those with a mental illness. We empathise with those who are suffering]

Before a patient reaches the extremes of chronic emotional stress, much can be done with regards the recovering of an emotional tone which is appropriate for the circumstances. To this end, Emotional Intelligence may be strengthened, whereby activation or inactivation is not experienced continuously, but tense or relaxed states are adapted, pertinent to the circumstances of each moment.

An appropriate therapeutic intervention, sometimes in conjunction with controlled pharmacological treatment can help the person recover their normal life, and, along with it, the social, family and partner relationships which, during their illness have suffered so much. The individual is therefore able to regain a suitable state of mind which allows for feelings of happiness.

However, happiness may be hindered by other feelings such as guilt, an emotion of which we are aware, which arises when we know that something wrong has been done, or that something which should have been done has not been. Therefore, guilt manifests itself as a feeling of blame regarding the undertaking (or not) of certain actions. In order for such feelings to arise the person must have a certain level of morality, or at least awareness of the fact that either what is being done does not meet socially desired expectations, or that a lack of action would be similarly undesirable

Currently it is understood that feelings of guilt, like pain, may be either positive or negative. For example, pain serves as a warning that all is not well in the body, and a 'remedy' must be found to alleviate it, this would be the 'positive' pain, whereas the 'negative' is when the pain continues over a period of time, even when measures have been taken to remedy it. So exactly the same thing happens with guilt, it is activated when something has been done which is known to be morally wrong, or something that should have happened does not. This should lead the individual to reflect upon why it was wrong and to try and remedy it as far as they are able, with the intention of not making the same mistake again once the 'lesson has been learned'. This may thus be seen as something positive, involving how an individual grows by learning from their mistakes. The negative element arises when the feelings of guilt remain for too long, even when a 'remedy' has been actioned in respect of its origins, and thus becomes an 'ordeal', making the individual feel bad within themself for something they cannot 'forget'.

People who suffer these 'stagnant' feelings of guilt, which will already form a part of their general demeanour, will experience various health problems, linked to this period of continuous stress, such as headache, stomach pain, tightness in the chest or tension in the shoulders. These people will also tend to exhibit the somewhat extremist way of 'thinking in black or white' where nuances of a situation are not appreciated, and they have intrusive thoughts of self-reproach and aggression towards themselves.

With regards negative guilt, three modes may be identified. Firstly, where the individual blames themself for 'all the evil in the world' whether it has anything to do with them or not. This is known as internal locus of control, whereby the individual believes that they are responsible for everything that happens around them, even though, in many instances, circumstances will not depend on the actions of the individual, but they are dependent upon the intervention of a third party.

The second position is whereby the blame for everything which happens to an individual is blamed on others, even if they have not participated in the act, and no responsibility is assumed by the individual. This is known as external locus of control, where someone else is blamed for anything that goes wrong, and it is usually adopted by 'immature' people who have remained at an earlier stage of moral development where they identify good with themselves and bad with others.

The third approach is where the individual excuses the responsibilities of both themself and others, by attributing everything to the circumstances of life, behaving as if they have agency to do whatsoever they please. Such is the defence used by people with few or low morals, in the sense that whatever they do they feel no responsibility for the results, and they will carry on doing exactly as they please. An example would be when an individual justifies themself by saying 'life made me this way' and does not bother to improve or change, continuing to do whatever they do with no sense of remorse.

In none of the aforementioned negative guilt positions does the individual attempt to analyse the circumstances which led to mistakes being made, nor is there any assumption of responsibility for the consequences that an action or inaction led to. Hence if the experience has not served as a lesson for the individual to reflect upon, the same mistake will be made the next time a similar situation arises.

Each of the above three situations will do nothing but harm the normal development of an individual, generating conflict wherever they may be, whether in the workplace or with a partner or family, since the feelings of guilt will be accompanied by a corresponding behaviour – in the first case of inactivity and avoiding outside contact so as to 'not do any more harm to the world', and in the second two cases simply seeking pleasure without looking any further. As in the case of frustration when expected goals are not achieved, this guilt will prevent the individual from enjoying a state of happiness, therefore they will first have to 'fix' their emotions in order to be free to search for happiness.

However, when talking about a population of millions confined to their homes, who thinks about happiness? As strange as it may seem, not only is it possible, but it is also quite fitting not to be focussing exclusively on the negative aspects of the current circumstances. Hence the government has changed their television programming schedule to include humorous slots, even making comic programmes about the current situation in order to make the lockdown situation more bearable for everyone. (@RTVE_Com, 2020) (See Illustration 36).

For years there has been talk of the benefits of being a positive person, particularly in the social sphere, although sometimes this particular term is confused with that of an optimist, since whereas positivity refers to a type of thought, optimism is a characteristic of personality.

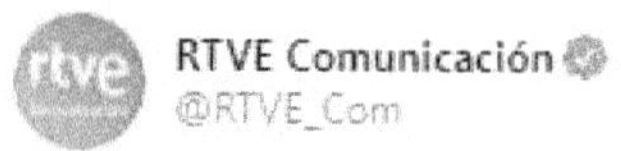

¡Llega 'Diarios de la cuarentena', una sitcom realista e íntima sobre el lado más divertido de la convivencia en tiempos de pandemia!

Estreno (y risas aseguradas) el martes a las 22:05 h en @La1_tve

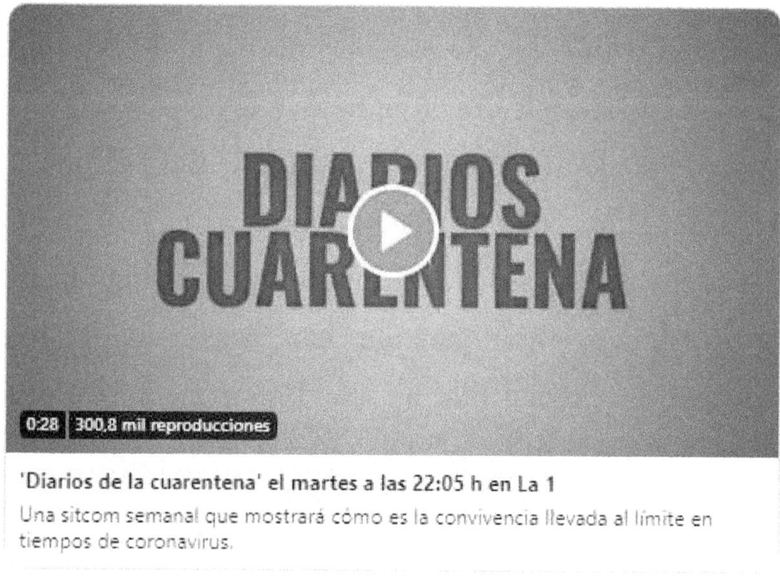

Illustration 36. Tweet – Humour in Lockdown

["Diarias de la cuarantena" (Diaries from Lockdown) has arrived. A realistic and revealing sitcom about the funniest side of living together in times of a pandemic]

Positive thoughts are those which make us appreciate what we have around us, where we feel that everything will go well, and that our efforts will be rewarded. Similarly, positive thinking allows us to believe that others will be fair and consistent in their judgements. Contrasting with these thoughts are the negative ones, where everything is horrible, unfair and inadequate and feelings of envy, self-criticism and lack of self-esteem are prioritised.

One type of thinking or another will tend to play a fundamental role in how others perceive and react to us, hence positive people are often held in high- esteem, whilst negative people are often 'marginalised' and left out. For this reason, it is socially more 'profitable' to be positive. But what is the role of positive thinking in the field of health? The answer to this question has been sought in an investigation carried out by the Department of Special Education, University of Thessaly (Greece) (Karampas, Michael & Stalikas, 2016).

The study involved 395 cadets from the Hellenic Army Academy aged between 18 and 22 years, of whom 123 were women. They all completed a standardised questionnaire in the evaluation of resilience – the Connor Davidson Resilience Scale (Connor & Davidson, 2003); another to evaluate positive thoughts – the Positive and Negative Affect Schedule (Watson, Clark & Tellegen, 1988); and one to assess general health via the General Health Questionnaire-28 (Goldberg & Hiller, 1979).

The results reported a significant correlation between positive thinking and resilience, i.e. the more positive thoughts a person has the more capability they feel in overcoming any obstacles in life. Equally significant correlations were obtained between positive thoughts and overall health, i.e. positive people were healthier than those with negative thoughts.

It should be taken into account that this study was undertaken with a very specific population - army cadets, who tend to be subjected to much higher levels of stress and demand than the rest of the population, so with that proviso in mind, it may be assumed that positive thinking serves to prevent illness amongst people subjected to high levels of pressure and anxiety. In the instances of those confined to their homes, although such a situation would not, initially be considered stressful, since people are at home, with their own belongings and their loved ones, the uncertainty as to when it will end, along with the health crisis itself, makes it a stressful and burdensome situation for some.

It is not being suggested that positive thinking may serve to combat COVID-19 or mitigate its effects if one is infected, but it does mean it can help in maintaining a better general state of health overall, an aspect which, along with healthy eating is emphasised by the health authorities as key in strengthening one's defences. Therefore, if the body does have to face the disease, it can do so under the best possible conditions.

One of the most frequent problems seen in the field of psychological consultation concerns emotions, either due to their over-activation, as in the case of stress and anxiety, or their inhibition, in the cases of sadness and depression. This is not because people are more sensitive to these problems and visit a psychologist more often, but rather that they are the most common mental health problems, experienced more than any other disorder in the field of mental health.

Sadness, along with happiness and fear, is considered to be one of the basic emotions, a state in which an individual no longer feels 'fulfilled' or even 'normal'. There are many reasons which can generate sadness, from the loss of a loved one to not having achieved a desired goal, but perhaps the most serious is the presence of a disease, especially if it is chronic or incurable.

The relationship between physical and mental health has long since ceased to be disputed. When someone suffers a disabling physical health condition this will have a direct effect both on their mood and in other areas, including the manner in which they relate to themselves and others.

When one feels bad, for instance when suffering from a chronic illness, this can significantly alter one's mood, even leading to depression. But when the symptoms of depression appear the situation gets worse, as the effect they have on health is important, reducing the quality of life of the individual by lowering not only the mood but also the immune system, placing the patient in a vicious circle. The worse they are physically the worse they feel psychologically, and the more depressive symptoms they suffer the worse their body will respond, therefore recovery, instead of being facilitated is hindered.

The consequences of such a vicious circle are an aggravation of the symptoms, worsening the patient's quality of life, making them less tolerant of what happens to them, and resulting in a worse prognosis for them than in another individual who has no depressive symptoms. It is therefore important for the first symptoms of depression to be diagnosed so they can be treated as soon as possible and do not progress and damage the health of the patient any further.

The origins of depression may be distinguished between exogenous and endogenous. Exogenous depression is caused by external 'negative' events experienced by the sufferer which affect their mood, e.g. the break-up of a relationship or the loss of a loved one, when the sadness felt extends beyond the usual mourning period.

Amongst the characteristic effects of depression are

feelings of guilt, hopelessness and futility, along with negative thoughts. In addition, there may be increased sensitivity to pain, persistent malaise, digestive problems, fatigue, irritability, indifference to previous interests, difficulty in concentration, and altered sleep patterns (too much or too little).

Although, as commented earlier, the relationship between physical and psychological health is long established, new discoveries are still being made. To date it has been known that when the body is 'mistreated' with too much pressure, wear and tear is caused and the body may 'fail' prematurely. This has been confirmed in studies since the 1960s when the term Type A personality emerged, defining those individuals who are particularly competitive and restless with high levels of stress and anxiety in their daily lives. In these people it was found that they were more likely to suffer from cardiac disease such as a heart attack which, if it occurs, not only increases the possibility of another one, but also significantly weakens this important muscle, and in many cases can shorten a person's life by months or even years.

In contrast, the term Type B personality emerged and was identified as being somewhat more protected from health issues and characterised by a calm individual with peace of mind who is governed by the values of cooperation and creativity, yet equally effective in the tasks they have to carry out. In this personality type the heart, far from being affected by the 'challenges' of the everyday, seems to be protected and there are fewer heart attacks than in those with Type A personality. But what happens with people who suffer with depression? This question has been addressed by a study undertaken by the School of Experimental Psychology, University of Bristol (UK) (Thomson, 2014).

The study involved 1413 participants of whom 785 had suffered depression (480 endogenous and 205 reactive). Their average ages were 44 for those who had suffered reactive (exogenous) depression and 58 for those who had suffered endogenous depression. More than half (67.7%) the participants were women. As a control group, data from the National Health Service Registry (England) was used, where information was obtained regarding the number of heart attacks suffered, and the survival rate of people in the same age groups.

The results found that men tend to suffer a significant shortening of life due to heart problems, but this relationship only occurred in the cases of endogenous depression.

There is depression currently being caused due to lockdown due to the temporary 'loss' for some people of activities which previously 'enriched' their emotional life, although based on previous research this will not pose a threat in terms of a shortening of life. However, attention must still be paid to emotional states, since they may well be influenced by the current lockdown situation, resulting in the appearance of anxiety and depression (@LANACION,2020) (See Illustration 37).

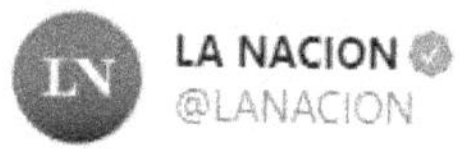

Coronavirus: uno de cada tres argentinos siente depresión y ansiedad por la cuarentena dlvr.it/RSs5m5

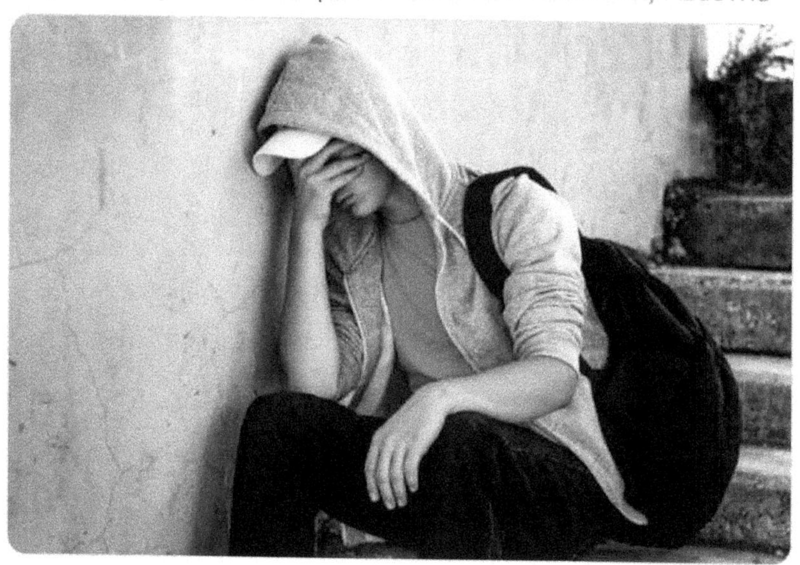

10:42 p. m. · 30 mar. 2020 · dlvr.it

Illustration 37. Tweet – Depression in Lockdown

[Coronavirus: one in three Argentinians feel depressed and anxious due to lockdown]

There are numerous situations throughout the day which require close attention. If a person is rushed or has too many demands at the same time, this can result in stress, which may manifest itself in the alteration of usual sleep patterns, causing insomnia.

Stress maintained in the medium to long term can be harmful to health, in what is known as distress. However, there also exists 'good' stress, the type which, for a short period of time enhances both capacity and responses to the task in hand. This type of stress is called eustress.

Whether stress is 'good' or 'bad' depends both upon the psychological assessment of stressful events and situations, as well as the length of time for which they persist. For instance, a situation viewed as challenging but appealing in the manner of improving oneself or 'showing off' will motivate the individual to give their best, thus obtaining success which otherwise would not have been achieved. However, if that same situation is maintained over time, a depletion of resources occurs, as explained in General Adaptation Syndrome (Selye, 1946) and the situation ceases to be motivating but instead becomes something 'insufferable' hence the stress takes over and wins. This syndrome divides stressful situations into three stages.

The initial stage is the alarm reaction where the organism prepares to respond to the stimulus or stressful situation.

The second stage of resistance or Adaptation is when the hypothalamic pituitary adrenal (HPA) mechanism is activated in response to the stressful demand. If the demand disappears a 'deactivation' process occurs via the same

HPA pathway, whereby the cortisol of the adrenal glands inhibits the production of the corticotropin-releasing hormone from the pituitary gland, which deactivates the HPA axis and recovers the basal levels prior to the onset of stress. On the other hand, if the stressful situation continues, the organism will continue to the next stage.

The final stage is exhaustion, based on the fact that the body's resources are limited and only available for a short time, and they eventually burn-out. This exhaustion brings a whole series of consequences to the different systems involved which may then cause the individual to become ill.

Medium term stress tends to lead to a series of consequences such as muscle aches, sleep and mood disturbances and immunodeficiency. Chronic stress, on the other hand, has more serious effects and may be responsible for digestive disorders leading to ulcers and diarrhoea; obesity due to increased appetite thus an increased risk of diabetes; weakening of the immune system and higher susceptibility to colds and infections; loss of memory, motivation, sleep, altered moods; increased blood pressure and heart rate; and accumulation of cholesterol and triglycerides in the blood with associated increased risk of heart disease and strokes.

On a psychological level chronic stress may also increase the symptoms of certain disorders, such as schizophrenia, where the higher the stress levels, the greater the expression of psychotic symptoms. In other people, the acute toxicity of high levels of cortisol in the brain affect certain neuronal structures leading to worsened cognitive performance. One such structure is the hippocampus, which is necessary for the establishment of new learning.

The immune system, which protects the body from internal and external infections, is very sensitive to emotional changes, particularly stress. When stress is generated the body will experience immunosuppression, reducing the use of these functions to a minimum, but if the stress is maintained the system will be damaged.

The first indications that the immune system is not working properly may be observed when symptoms of conditions such as psoriasis or lupus appear. If no remedy is found and the stressful situation continues, there will not only be a slowdown in the healing and recovery process of any existing conditions, but the door is 'left open' to all kinds of other infections, as well as producing a worsening of any autoimmune diseases such as multiple sclerosis.

The HPA axis, when functioning correctly, produces a timely activation in the body in stressful situations, allowing an individual to give the right response at the right moment, whether it be of 'fight or flight'. However, if this activation is maintained over time, because the cause of stress is still present, 'malfunctions' occur in the normal processes, thereby increasing the likelihood for the individual to suffer from various diseases. This is due to the close relationship between the immune and psychological systems, the former being responsible for the correct recovery of any disorder within the organism, and low defences not only slow down this process, but also contribute to the onset of infections and other diseases. As mentioned previously, this relationship is also mediated by personality factors, with Type A and Type B personalities connected with higher and lower levels of heart disease respectively.

It is therefore known that high levels of stress will mainly affect the health of the heart, and that those with Type A personality are more likely to suffer health attacks than those with Type B personality. These two personality types are the most well-known, although a few years ago two other types were discovered, Type C and D.

In Type C personality there is a high level of expression of emotion, particularly positive ones. The individual tends to be very positive, hiding their negative emotions from others. They tend to suffer from rheumatism, infections, skin allergies, skin diseases and cancer.

Individuals with Type D personality, which is perhaps the least well-known type, exhibit a high level of self-demand, with hyperactive behaviour and low self -esteem and disconnection between the emotional and the 'rational' world, making them more likely to suffer form psychosomatic diseases. Ulcerative colitis, peptic ulcers and vascular disorders such as hypertension are also more likely to occur in this personality type.

The same lockdown situation will therefore have different effects on moods, emotions and the immune system for each individual, dependent upon their personality type. Type B personality seems to be the type most associated with a satisfactory state of general health, due to the calm manner in which they approach life's challenges, considering them to be transient circumstances which must be lived through, but which cause no increase in anxiety, thus stress and its effects are avoided.

Although in times of lockdown measures have been put in place by governments ensuring that all its citizens have access to food, it should be taken into account that one's state of mind will always influence the choice of what is eaten, in quantity as well as quality.

Suffering depressive symptoms, together with the loss of interest in something which previously gave pleasure (anhedonia) can make the individual, little by little 'abandon' certain elements, such as personal hygiene and nutrition. There is an increase in the consumption of high calorie foods and alcohol, causing weight changes and, if accompanied by binge eating as a way to 'fill' one's life, this can cause weight gain which may eventually lead to obesity.

However, depression may also cause the opposite effect, i.e. the 'bad' diet leads to weight loss. In this instance the diet, coupled with lack of sleep, which means being awake more hours of the day (characteristic of people with depression) means the individual is active, hence burning more calories, but in this particular instance the calories are not being replaced due to the inadequate diet.

For some years there has been evidence of a close relationship between depression and obesity, with a greater number of obese people suffering from depression and, equally, people suffering from depression have a higher percentage of obesity. It is not clear, however, whether it is depression which is the cause of obesity or vice versa.

It must be borne in mind that obese people tend to be more susceptible to teasing from others, especially at an early age. They are particularly sensitive in the pre-adolescent phase, when the opinion and judgement of others is of paramount importance. For a young person, being rejected or ridiculed can act as a trigger, undermining their self-esteem, which may lead to isolation and the avoidance of social relationships. At the same time, they may 'retreat' into food,

using it as a way of 'filling up' on the love they lack.

A study analysing the effects on depression of an intervention on obesity was carried out by the Department of Psychology, Faculty of Humanities, Bond University; The Lakeside Rooms Centre, and the Mullumbimby Psychology Centre (Australia) together with the Foundation for Epigenetic Medicine (USA) (Stapleton, Church, Sheldon, Porter & Carlopio, 2013).

The study consisted of 96 obese adult participants, half of whom were given an Emotional Freedom Technique (Church, 2017) treatment, while the rest did not carry out any form of treatment. The four-week treatment directly intervened on obesity, whilst with regards the depressive symptoms, an evaluation was carried out before and after treatment to see if they had been affected, and if so, to what extent.

The results showed positive effects, both in terms of reduction in obesity and improvement of depressive symptoms, effects which were maintained over time, as confirmed by results from an assessment twelve months later.

The above results confirm the positive effects of the intervention both on obesity and depression, allowing a general rethink on the way in which major depressive disorder is treated, avoiding the side effects in some patients of a drug- based intervention treatment, whether presented in isolation or in combination with psychotherapy.

It is known that, once childhood is over, in which there are more sleeping than waking hours in a day, that proportion is reversed, and the body requires around eight hours sleep per day for the rest of its life. This schedule may not always be maintained, resulting in some losses and some accumulations of sleep during certain periods which will subsequently be recovered. For instance, the working day is longer in the shifts of some jobs, or young people may stay up late studying or partying, and they will eventually compensate for this 'accumulation' with a long sleep.

Similarly, it is natural in the elderly for sleep time to be split, and instead of sleeping eight hours in a row, they tend to wake up after the first five hours, completing the remaining three hours a few hours later. But even in the elderly there is a tendency to abandon this type of 'fragmented' sleep, and there is often a kind of 'deregulation' where microsleeps are taken, regardless of what time it is, since they do not recognise that proper sleep is essential for the proper functioning of the brain, even when elderly.

Whilst discussing the importance of sleep, it requires mention that in the event of an accumulation of sleepless nights, e.g. in the studying for an exam or working of night shifts, the effects will become increasingly significant and serious, affecting both physical and psychological health and social relationships. Physically, muscle mass will decrease, along with an increased tendency to suffer illnesses, since the immune system reaches peak activity during sleep. Furthermore, injuries caused by lack of attention and increased possibility of accidents will occur. On a psychological level, there is a reduction in attention and concentration and inability to focus. With regards social relationships, others will realise and react accordingly. Furthermore, excess fatigue will either result in sufferers not wishing to spend time with others and, if they do, they may be irritable, ultimately resulting in loss of social contacts.

Classic experiments regarding sleep deprivation demonstrate devastating effects on attention, performance and other cognitive functions such as learning. Sleep deprivation may also put the mental health of an individual at risk who, after days without sleep becomes exhausted, drained and irritable, with moments of euphoria, paranoid thoughts, and subject to psychotic episodes, all due to not sleeping well.

Similarly, sleep deprivation has an important effect on decision-making, according to the study carried out by the

Sleep Research Centre of Loughborough University (UK) (Horne, 2012). This has also been evidenced by experiments concerning decision-making with regard to future profits as, for example, in the Iowa Gambling Task (Buelow & Suhr, 2009) which demonstrates the accuracy of decisions taken, based on variables set by the experimenter, who manipulates the amount of possible gains or losses in each trial.

There are four tasks with possible established results of high gain, small gain, small loss or high loss. Once a baseline measurement on performance is obtained, the tasks are performed again after some hours of sleep deprivation, usually 24 hours, in order to observe the interference or not of lack of sleep in the decisions taken.

Research suggests that deprivation of 49 hours sleep causes the participants to take risky decisions such as would be taken by individuals with injuries to the ventral prefrontal cortex. These studies were undertaken by the Division of Neuropsychiatry, Walter Reed Armed Forces Research Institute ; Maryland Psychiatric Research Center; Department of Psychiatry, University of Maryland; Department of Radiology of the School of Medicine, and the Department of Environmental Health Sciences of the School of Public Health and Hygiene, John Hopkins Institute of Medicine (USA) together with the Rotman

Research Institute and University of Toronto (Canada) (Colten & Altevogt, 2006).

It may therefore be concluded that lack of sleep not only reduces cognitive abilities, affects emotionality, and impedes the immune system, but also leads a person to make 'bad' decisions, hence the importance of maintaining a regular sleep pattern of at least eight hours per night.

When speaking about the role of stress in the emotional world and its consequences on the organism, reference must be made to the term of resilience, which has become a key psychological concept in recent years, referring to the manner in which a person copes with life.

The term resilience arose from the testimony of survivors of some of the most extreme situations to which people can be subjected, such as the Nazi concentration camps in World War Two. It was analysed as to why, despite living through the same horrific circumstances of war, some had survived and others not, and why some of the survivors managed to rebuild their lives, yet others were plunged into despair.

This analysis, and testimonies such as that of Victor Frankl, who developed logotherapy as a method of dealing with such situations (Frankl, 2004) led to the emergence of this kind of formula of overcoming any adversity, something which appears to be linked to a person's character, as well as their way of thinking and seeing life. This concept is currently used in therapy, not only in helping those who have survived extreme situations, but in helping people overcome the daily difficulties of life, aiming at reinforcing the resilience which everyone has inside them.

Resilience is therefore a concept which may be learned and developed, and which has a critical role to play in protecting the individual, since everyone is exposed to stress on a daily basis. With development of resilience it is possible to learn how to overcome any difficulties which may arise, and it is therefore important that it is taught to children at an early age.

The boom in the eighties within the field of Emotional Psychology and, more specifically, within its applied branch of Emotional Intelligence, has resulted in a rather specific vocabulary, which may not be familiar to everyone. Included in this vocabulary is the term of resilience, which may be understood as the set of personal capacities and abilities available to the individual allowing them to face the most difficult situations and emerge victorious from them.

Although some have identified resilience as a personal quality with which one is born, rather like charisma, it is largely considered that it can be developed and improved, thus enabling one to have the necessary tools to cope with the challenges of everyday life, something which is essential in any job or profession. But from what age is it appropriate to learn about resilience? This question has been addressed by a study undertaken by the Faculty of

Science and Technology, Technological and Higher Education Institute of Hong Kong (Hong Kong) (Tung, Ning & Kris, 2014).

There were 257 participants in the study, all high school students, 86% of them between 16 and 20 years of age and the rest over 20 years of age, half of whom were girls. Each student was given a questionnaire to ascertain their levels of stress, whether there were physical symptoms associated with any stress, the presence of depression, and their levels of self-confidence, self-esteem and optimism.

The results reported that half of the participants considered they had

good levels of resilience, self-esteem and personal self-control. In terms of comparison according to gender, the girls demonstrated higher anxiety levels and lower social perception. Children from single parent families, who constituted 10% of the participants, showed lower levels of resilience and self-esteem as compared to the rest of their peers.

Evaluated overall, it can be concluded that the results are not a particular cause for concern. Whilst half of the students have low resilience which, as the authors suggest, may lead to sleep disorders associated with anxiety as well as other psychosomatic disorders, resilience can be learned and developed, and it is extremely useful in increasing self-esteem and academic performance.

It is therefore important that resilience be detected and developed from childhood, in order that the individual may be prepared for the day to day challenges they will face, whether at work or in their personal life. Resilience is essential when facing a situation such as that of lockdown where, due to the exceptional nature of the situation, high levels of stress may be generated, which can even lead to feelings of worthlessness and depression. As long as one knows how to put the situation in perspective and find a sense of 'meaning' in life, it will be much easier to face and cope with the situation.

List of Illustrations

Referenced Tweets

@ConsejoCOLEF. (2020). Consejo COLEF en Twitter: ".@deportegob y @ConsejoCOLEF recomiendan seguir manteniendo estilos de vida activos durante el confinamiento. Si tienes dudas sobre cómo entrenar en casa, contacta con profesionales cualificados/as del deporte. #YoMeMuevoEnCasa. Retrieved April 5, 2020, from https://twitter.com/ConsejoCOLEF/status/1245005430096646151

@diariodeburgos. (2020). Diario de Burgos en Twitter: "Hoy en DB: El virus destruye en Burgos en 15 días el empleo creado en 2 años 2 detenidos y más de 600 multas por saltarse el confinamiento Bajan un 70% las urgencias desde el coronavirus Infantil y Primaria pierden otros mil. Retrieved April 5, 2020, from https://twitter.com/diariodeburgos/status/1245946653867151361

@LANACION. (2020). LA NACION en Twitter: "Coronavirus: uno de cada tres argentinos siente depresión y ansiedad por la cuarentena https://t.co/CWVlbjUnrb https://t.co/OmPUUrydBh" / Twitter. Retrieved April 7, 2020, from https://twitter.com/LANACION/status/1244726615902269441

@ma_pureza. (2020). MaPureza en Twitter: "Hoy, en el Día Mundial del Trastorno Bipolar, hagamos conciencia sobre esta enfermedad. El aislamiento puede ser desafiante para muchos, pero es un reto para aquellos que tienen enfermedades mentales. Tengamos empatía con aquellos qu. Retrieved April 5, 2020, from https://twitter.com/ma_pureza/status/1244753247107272705

@RTVE_Com. (2020). RTVE Comunicación en Twitter: "?¡Llega "Diarios de la cuarentena", una sitcom realista e íntima sobre el lado más divertido de la convivencia en tiempos de pandemia! ? Estreno (y risas aseguradas) el martes a las 22:05 h en @La1_tve https://t.co/Gk34fN2. Retrieved April 5, 2020, from https://twitter.com/RTVE_Com/status/1245748325346918401

References

Bastian, B., Koval, P., Erbas, Y., Houben, M., Pe, M., & Kuppens, P. (2015). Sad and Alone. *Social Psychological and Personality Science*, *6*(5), 496–503. https://doi.org/10.1177/1948550614568682

Bhargawa, M. (2012). Dimensional Personality Inventory. *National Psychological Corporation, Agra.*

Buelow, M. T., & Suhr, J. A. (2009, March 5). Construct validity of the Iowa gambling task. *Neuropsychology Review*, Vol. 19, pp. 102–114. https://doi.org/10.1007/s11065-009-9083-4

Chandola, D. R. (2016). Is personality of schizophrenics & bipolar patients are similar? *International Journal of Sciences & Applied Research*, *3*(5), 51–59.

Church, D. (2017). *The EFT manual*. Hay House, Inc.

Colten, H. R., & Altevogt, B. M. (2006). Sleep disorders and sleep deprivation: An unmet public health problem. In *Sleep Disorders and Sleep Deprivation: An Unmet Public Health Problem*. https://doi.org/10.17226/11617

Connor, K. M., & Davidson, J. R. T. (2003). Development of a new Resilience scale: The Connor-Davidson Resilience scale (CD-RISC). *Depression and Anxiety*, *18*(2), 76–82. https://doi.org/10.1002/da.10113

Frankl, V. E. (2014). *The will to meaning: Foundations and applications of logotherapy*. Penguin.

Goldberg, D. P., & Hillier, V. F. (1979). A scaled version of the General Health Questionnaire. *Psychological Medicine*, *9*(1), 139–145. https://doi.org/10.1017/S0033291700021644

Horne, J. (2012, November 1). Working throughout the night: Beyond "sleepiness" - impairments to critical decision making. *Neuroscience and Biobehavioral Reviews*, Vol. 36, pp. 2226–2231. https://doi.org/10.1016/j.neubiorev.2012.08.005

Karampas, K., Michael, G., & Stalikas, A. (2016). Positive

Emotions, Resilience and Psychosomatic Heath: Focus on Hellenic Army NCO Cadets. *Psychology*, *07*(13), 1727–1740. https://doi.org/10.4236/psych.2016.713162

Luna, K. (2020). Speaking of Psychology: Coronavirus Anxiety. Retrieved February 29, 2020, from APA.org website: https://www.apa.org/research/action/speaking-of-psychology/coronavirus-anxiety

Pi, Y.-L., Wu, X.-H., Wang, F.-J., Liu, K., Wu, Y., Zhu, H., & Zhang, J. (2019). Motor skill learning induces brain network plasticity: A diffusion-tensor imaging study. *PLOS ONE*, *14*(2), e0210015. https://doi.org/10.1371/journal.pone.0210015

Radloff, L. S. (1977). The CES-D Scale: A Self-Report Depression Scale for Research in the General Population. *Applied Psychological Measurement*, *1*(3), 385–401. https://doi.org/10.1177/014662167700100306

Russell, D. W. (1996). UCLA Loneliness Scale (Version 3): Reliability, validity, and factor structure. *Journal of Personality Assessment*, *66*(1), 20–40. https://doi.org/10.1207/s15327752jpa6601_2

Selye, H. (1946). The General Adaptation Syndrome and the Diseases of Adaptation. *The Journal of Clinical Endocrinology & Metabolism*, *6*(2), 117–230. https://doi.org/10.1210/jcem-6-2-117

Stapleton, P., Church, D., Sheldon, T., Porter, B., & Carlopio, C. (2013). Depression symptoms improve after successful weight loss with emotional freedom techniques. *ISRN Psychiatry*, *2013*, 573532. https://doi.org/10.1155/2013/573532

Thomson, W. (2014). The Head Stands Accused by the Heart! —Depression and Premature Death from Ischaemic Heart Disease. *Open Journal of Depression*, *03*(02), 33–40. https://doi.org/10.4236/ojd.2014.32008

Tung, K. S., Ning, W. W., & Kris, L. T. Y. A. (2014). Effect of Resilience on Self-Perceived Stress and Experiences on Stress Symptoms A Surveillance Report. *Universal*

Journal of Public Health, *2*(2), 64–72. https://doi.org/10.13189/UJPH.2014.020205

Watson, D., Clark, L. A., & Tellegen, A. (1988). Development and Validation of Brief Measures of Positive and Negative Affect: The PANAS Scales. *Journal of Personality and Social Psychology*, *54*(6), 1063–1070. https://doi.org/10.1037/0022-3514.54.6.1063

Conclusions

This work attempts to give a scientifically researched perspective on an exceptional situation, as in the case of the health crisis currently being experienced.

There have been many recommendations and good advice offered on this subject, in most cases based on personal experiences. This work offers an alternative vision, from the science of psychology, containing results of research carried out throughout the world, in an effort to support and help at this particular time.

www.ingramcontent.com/pod-product-compliance
Ingram Content Group UK Ltd.
Pitfield, Milton Keynes, MK11 3LW, UK
UKHW021910190726
13853UKWH00002B/603